DON'T DIE EARLY:

THE LIFE YOU SAVE CAN BE YOUR OWN

Don't Die Early:

The Life You Save Can Be Your Own

Rocky Angelucci

LRA Publishing, LLC
McKinney, Texas
USA

Published in the United States of America by LRA Associates, LLC.
5100 Eldorado Parkway #102-365
McKinney, TX 75070

ISBN 978-0-9854045-0-5

First LRA Associates edition, third printing. Published 2012.

www.dontdieearly-book.com

Dedication

To Laura and Sophia.

Disclaimer

I'm not a doctor. I'm not trying to be your doctor and you shouldn't try and be your own doctor, either. What you should be is *your own greatest medical advocate.*

This book is for informational purposes only. It is not intended to be medical advice. Make no changes to your diet, exercise regimen, medications, or nutritional supplements without consulting your healthcare provider.

And finally, despite my mentioning a number of suppliers, online communities, and vendors throughout this book, I have received no compensation of any kind from them. Neither do any of them endorse what I have said here. They are just sources of goods and services that have served me well, but as the saying goes, "Your mileage may vary."

CONTENTS

ACKNOWLEDGMENTS

I want to thank those people without whom this book would have not been possible, or if it did happen, it would have taken far longer and been much less impressive.

First, thank you to my wife Laura, who started this whole thing with "You really need to write a book about this." I'm not certain she realized the implications of being someone's muse and in doing so, subjecting herself to the whiplash-inducing mix of "leave me alone, I'm busy!" and "come quick, I need your help!" Her tireless support in this project, and in all things, is invaluable to me. And to Sophia, who had to hear, "not now, I'm working on my book" way more often than any little girl should endure.

My reviewers, Barbie Anderson, Laura Angelucci, Gary Henson, Royce Herndon, Carley Phillips, Louise Phillips PhD, and Toni Poster, helped turn semi-coherent emails and notes into an organized manuscript.

Jay Angelucci, Erica Olenski, and Jeff Zinger taught me about life on the web, including the difference between *twitter* and *twaddle* and between *facebook* and *faceplant.*

And to my proofreader, Leslie Phillips, and editor Jill Kelly PhD, for toning down my excessively passionate rage against the status quo.

Thank you to Laura Angelucci for her cover design assistance. And to whoever's feet those are in the picture, I'm sorry this book didn't come soon enough to help you.

And thank you to Dr. N. Christopher Lawrence for suggesting the title, *Don't Die Early,* which captures my intent perfectly.

FOREWORD

by N. Christopher Lawrence, MD

Fear, usually accompanied by a desire to flee or fight, I imagine, is what Rocky Angelucci felt that day in March 2010 as he experienced a life-changing cardiac event that began his journey to write this powerful book about change. No one needs to die early because of poor choices of diet and exercise, or the lack of the knowledge to prevent. I have had the inspiring privilege of watching Rocky pursue his own quest for wellness. Rocky represents all people. A normal guy, living a normal life, that one day changes, in his case for the better. This will not be the case for everyone...

Don't die early.

As a family physician for 17 years, I have enjoyed serving countless patients on their quest to a healthy life. As a traditionally trained MD, however, I was taught to prescribe medication for high blood pressure, high cholesterol, diabetes, depression, and all other diseases of our bodies. I have since learned to call this "Band-Aid" medicine. Putting a Band-Aid on a problem does not cure the problem. Covering up an issue with a Band-Aid only delays the progression to a worsened issue. I was never taught at a formal level the idea of true wellness and disease prevention at the level of the entire body.

For the last 7 years I have been researching and learning about functional medicine, a form of Western alternative medicine that focuses on treating patients who have imbalances, symptoms, and dysfunctions. It seeks to identify the root cause of disease and views the body as one system, not a collection of organs divided up by medical specialties. To treat the body as a complex system and to be aware of how all parts affect the others can provide a framework to provide a more comprehensive style of healthcare to our patients. We can help our patients prevent and cure disease, not just treat symptoms so that they can live with disease.

Don't Die Early sets up a remarkable framework as a tool of wellness to help guide better choices and inform those at risk of disease to pursue a more aggressive approach to their healthcare. Doctors are busy, they are system-oriented, and they frequently do not see the big picture or are unwilling to think outside of the box. But it is your life that is at stake, you have to take control.

Don't Die Early is a plan of wellness and longevity. If you want to live free of disease and the risk of disease, you must begin to make changes in your diet, your level of exercise, in the toxicity of your environment, and in the levels of stress. We have the tools that we need; we must be wise enough to use them. Rocky Angelucci, just a regular guy writing a life-changing book about change, has set the foundation and given you the knowledge to go about changing your future. Please read, listen, and act. Don't die early...

N. Christopher Lawrence, MD

Board Certified Family Physician in McKinney, Texas

My Story

Lying on the gurney in the emergency room, I shielded my eyes from the glaring overhead lights and tried to remember exactly when my heart went wacko.

I remember being anxious and out of sorts all evening. Looking back, I realized that during dinner my chest felt fluttery and strange inside, and I recall snapping at my wife, Laura, over nothing as I left the kitchen to go upstairs.

By the time I reached the top of the stairs, I knew something was very wrong—I could barely breathe and when I placed my fingers to the side of my neck, my pulse felt very unusual. Not the rhythmic beating I would have expected, but more like an indistinct, squishy fluttering. Walking into our spare bedroom, I retrieved the pulse meter from the shelf next to the treadmill. I slipped the meter on my finger and looked at the readout. The effort seemed exhausting. Sitting on the edge of the bed, I called for Laura. When she arrived a moment later, I handed her the pulse meter.

The display read 195 beats per minute and I knew my life had just changed forever. The old carefree way of taking care of my body that had worked fine in my youth and young adulthood wasn't working anymore. I now had to become a conscious advocate of my own health.

The past two years have been an amazing journey for me. Through a great deal of research and persistence, I turned the vague intention to *be healthier* into a clear definition of what *healthier* meant to me and significantly improved my condition in every measurable way.

In the first six months after embracing a preventive lifestyle, I accomplished the following:

- Lowered my body fat percentage from 20% to 11%
- Lowered my inflammatory markers by as much as 75% (you'll learn about inflammation later)
- Reduced my triglycerides by more than 90% (this happened in the first 30 days)
- Improved every measurable aspect of my cholesterol
- Improved my fasting glucose by 25%
- Improved my muscle tone and stamina
- Lowered my blood pressure from an average of 145/90 to an average of 115/70
- Reduced my resting heart rate by more than 13 points

As impressive as these results might appear, I'm not revealing them so that you'll invite me to your next party. They are to show you what is very attainable for anyone who makes the proper lifestyle changes.

While the effort required to *achieve* these goals wasn't herculean, *defining* the goals took a great deal more work, largely because of the conflicting information available today about what's healthy and what's not.

My first step after returning home from the hospital was to learn more about the atrial fibrillation that took me there.[1] The hospital cardiologist used the phrase "once a fibber, always a fibber" to mean that once a person experiences an episode of atrial fibrillation (a-fib), the a-fib will reappear for the rest of a person's life. My

1. The biggest danger of atrial fibrillation is the formation of blood clots in the poorly beating heart, possibly leading to a stroke.

research indicated that this isn't always the case, with most adults today being deficient in magnesium and potassium, deficiencies of which are believed to cause atrial fibrillation, coupled with an excess of calcium, also common among adults today. (I had little trouble believing that low magnesium played a role in atrial fibrillation because magnesium was the first thing the physician attached to my IV when I arrived at the ER.)

After vowing to increase my magnesium and potassium intake to thwart any future a-fib events, I turned my attention to coronary artery disease, a condition that's common in my family history. For some reason, the cardiologist's statement that the stress echocardiogram he had performed would show blockages as small as 15% didn't sound right to me.[1] It didn't take long to learn that the cardiologist's assurance was off by more than a factor of five—a stress echo doesn't typically show blockages until an artery is 70–80% blocked. Not only had I discovered a number of cardiologists and other practitioners asserting this 70–80% figure, I found an alarming number of testimonials from people who passed a stress test and yet required an angioplasty, stent, or bypass within a year or less.

Learning about the shortcomings of a stress test caused my feelings of uncertainty to grow. If the cardiologist could be so wrong about the value of a stress test, what other misconceptions were being propagated by well-meaning, yet possibly misinformed, practitioners?

One thing that seemed certain was the danger of my elevated triglycerides. Days of research confirmed that elevated triglycerides contribute directly to coronary artery disease and that the most likely culprits for my elevated triglycerides were carbohydrates (with fructose being especially effective at elevating triglycerides). This, and a fasting glucose that was closer to 100 mg/dL than I cared to admit, prompted my first dietary change: lowering my carbohydrate intake. I immediately eliminated all wheat, rice, corn, potatoes, processed sugar, and fruit juices from my diet, replacing them with vegetables, nuts, and berries.

---

1. A *stress echo* is a combination stress test and echocardiogram, in which the heart is stressed, either by using a treadmill or through medication; it uses ultrasound to study the heart's performance.

Thirty-five days later, I checked my triglycerides again and saw that they had dropped from 1,193 mg/dL to 117, a 90% reduction. My other lab results improved dramatically, as well, and were clearly on the way to the values that I described above. This compelled me to learn even more and try even harder.

By now, I had also learned that the standard cholesterol test is not very useful in determining if we're likely to be producing cardiac plaque. I found a physician who knew all about more advanced ways of testing lipids and I gathered some baseline data so that I could objectively measure my continued progress. While the best time for this advanced lipid analysis would have been before I made *any* changes, I was still happy to have them one month into my new lifestyle. I had also learned a great deal about inflammation and its role in heart disease, diabetes, and autoimmune diseases and vowed to start taking steps to reduce my inflammation.

Permeating all of my research into cardiovascular health and inflammation was the importance of blood glucose control, even for those of us who would never think of using words like *insulin* or *diabetic*. Buying a glucose meter and studying the effects of certain foods on my blood glucose was eye-opening, to say the least. By removing wheat, rice, corn, potatoes, processed sugar, and fruit juices from my diet, I was seeing my fasting glucose level begin to drop, a clear sign that insulin resistance was improving. My diet was best defined at this time by the term *paleo*, a philosophy that embraces eating foods that our hunter-gatherer ancestors ate: lean meats, vegetables, nuts, and berries. Even though *paleo* is still the best category into which I can place my diet, I've made some subtle changes due to specific aspects of my physiology.

For the next year or so, I used objective laboratory testing and measurement to refine my diet and my supplements, to zero in on the optimum lifestyle for me. As I'm fond of saying, no matter what one study or another says, nothing will tell you the effects of lifestyle changes like objective testing will. It was during this time I learned a great deal about scientific journals, types of research studies, statistics, and the difference between science and marketing (and just how blurry the line between the two can be). I emerged from this far more equipped to spot the subtle and not so subtle ways in which news headlines, advertising, and research can be distorted to achieve a specific goal.

The path from that fateful night in the ER to where I am today was by no means simple and it was very frustrating at times. By learning what I've learned, however, you'll be much better equipped to accurately assess your health and chart a path towards improved health.

About This Book

It's a mess out there. Obesity, diabetes, heart disease, and inflammatory diseases are all on the rise. And it seems that everyone has answers. We are bombarded daily by an endless torrent of ads for healthy foods, weight loss clinics, medications, and medical practitioners, all promising to make us healthier. Yet we seem to be getting less and less healthy all the time.

How does a person know what's right and what's wrong? How do we separate fact from carefully crafted half-truths? Making the answers more difficult are the differences between us as individuals, meaning that some things are right for virtually everyone while other things vary considerably from person to person.

When I left the emergency room in March 2010, I began seeking answers. Digging into countless books, blogs, websites, research publications, and user forums, I started asking hard questions about what defines good health and what lifestyle decisions were required to achieve good health. Through it all I learned that a great deal of what is held as common knowledge is misunderstood, oversimplified, or just plain wrong.

I began putting what I had learned into practice, and soon my family and friends began asking how I had brought about the changes that were so easy for them to see. I found myself answering the same questions over and over again. I decided that the best thing to do was to write everything down once and make it available.

This book is a guide to identifying the biggest factors that affect our health today, to honestly assessing your condition, and to making lifestyle changes that can promote improved health, no matter your age or history.

I believe that by controlling certain aspects of our "care and feeding," we can reduce our risk of certain diseases, reduce some of the severity if we already have them, and generally improve the quality and possibly the duration of our life.

One of the biggest reasons that diabetes, heart disease, high blood pressure, and autoimmune diseases are so prevalent today is that the disease process begins long before the outward symptoms appear, yet we often wait until the disease has manifested itself before we take action. Despite it being contrary to human nature, a much more effective strategy is to start paying attention to preventive health while you still feel fine and while there's still time to make course corrections that will improve your health for the rest of your life. It's never too early to begin.

Part 1 explains how each of these health factors affects us, and dispels misinformation about each. What you'll also learn in Part 1 is that even if you've been told you are free from heart disease, have healthy cholesterol levels and little risk of diabetes, you may, in fact, be suffering from some or all of these without knowing it.

Chapter 1 defines coronary artery disease, discusses how to measure our risk and determining whether we have it, and addresses what it means if we do have heart disease. Chapter 2 presents a fundamental concept about coronary disease: cholesterol. These two chapters pave the way for addressing what to do in response to heart disease.

Chapter 3 looks at glucose control. I can almost hear you thinking, "I can certainly skip these chapters because I'm not diabetic." As with coronary artery disease, diabetes can sneak up on us, manifesting itself decades before traditional medical tests show that we're diabetic.

Chapter 4 brings us to inflammation. Far from an isolated event, however, inflammation is a continuous process carried out by the immune system and is a critical component of our body's repair and defense mechanisms. The problem arises when our lifestyle causes more inflammation than our immune system is designed to handle.

In Chapter 4 you'll learn that inflammation is far more rampant than most people realize and, in most cases, is caused primarily by our lifestyle choices, including things that the experts say are good for us.

Part 2 will discuss assessing our condition and specific goals and lifestyle changes that can help us improve our overall health.

Each chapter contains a summary of important points and actions you may wish to consider if you're inspired to act immediately. The final chapter ties theories and goals into a plan of action for you to consider.

Some people may start at the plan of action and read the preceding chapters later to better understand the justification behind it. Others may want the background and foundation first so that the plan of action makes logical sense in the context of what they're learned. Some people may want to skip around, reading chapters that sound interesting, before settling on a specific approach. How you take all this in is entirely up to you and there's no right or wrong way to go about it.

Read. Learn. Enjoy.

INTRODUCTION

- Do you think that even though there are some great doctors out there, *you* yourself are primarily responsible for maintaining your health?
- Do you enjoy rolling up your sleeves and learning about complex subjects?
- Do you prefer to adopt a healthy life to *prevent* disease and illness rather than live carelessly and hope that the doctors can keep you well?
- Do you believe that mainstream sources of medical information may be oversimplifying things and may not be getting everything right?
- Are you willing to challenge, or even disregard, common medical opinions if your research leads you to believe something else is true?

If you answered "yes" to most of these questions, then congratulations, you've found a great starting point!

MISCONCEPTIONS I HAD TO UNLEARN

The first time I drove a jet ski, I learned a good lesson. Years of driving a car had taught me that if I was trying to avoid an obstacle or make a quick turn, I needed to first let up on the gas pedal so that I could better maneuver the car. Applying this knowledge to the jet ski, however, proved disastrous, for this type of watercraft steers with jets of water and without the throttle, there's no steering. So I had to overcome intuition, ignore the little voice inside that's yelling "slow down, you're about to crash!" and apply lots of throttle while steering the craft away from an obstacle.

In other words, learning to drive a jet ski required that I first abandon what I had believed to be a fundamental truth: reducing velocity helps to control steering. Similarly, charting a path toward optimum health required that I abandon a number of concepts that I believed to be absolutely true. For example, I learned that:

- Being fit *doesn't* guarantee that you are healthy.
- Passing a cardiac stress test *is not* a trustworthy indication that you are safe from a heart attack or free of coronary artery disease.
- A standard lipid test tells you *very little* about how likely you are to be producing cardiac plaque.
- Being overweight *does not* simply mean that you eat more calories than you should.
- When your labs say you are "normal," it *doesn't* mean you are healthy.

ARE YOU WILLING TO WORK HARD FOR YOUR HEALTH?

Most of us go about our busy lives, believing that "the experts" have things in control. Sure, we may have some unhealthy habits or maybe we don't eat an optimal diet all the time and we probably should exercise a little bit more, but we basically live in a generally healthy manner, don't we?

If something feels wrong, we'll go to the doctor and if the physical and the cholesterol test we get every few years comes back okay, we know we're doing fine. We tell ourselves that this is as much as any reasonable person can do.

What I discovered is that this just isn't enough if you want to be as healthy as you can be. Being healthier takes a commitment to learning and making changes.

Although medicine is changing fast, because of the extremely cautious and measured way information flows from research to practice, research can be decades ahead of the advice you'll hear from your physician. It's therefore up to us to roll up our sleeves and become students of preventive health.

What Will Motivate You?

A friend whose opinion I respect advised me to make my book motivational, not just informative. Information is straightforward to find, he argued. It's motivation that many people find the hardest to muster.

While this seemed like sound advice, I have no idea how to motivate you to change. If the desire for a healthier life isn't sufficient motivation enough, what else will do it?

Because you want to be around as long as possible for your spouse or your children?

Because you don't want to spend the final decades of your life in horrible health, stagnating, while others your age are still enjoying life?

Only you can know.

For me, it's pretty simple. I want to avoid as many of the diseases that are plaguing our society as possible. I don't want to have a heart attack or a stroke and I don't want to get cancer. I want to spend my years living life as fully as possible, not staring at a wall in a nursing home. While it certainly may come to that, I'd prefer it to be as late in my life as possible.

One tool I've found useful in examining my own motivations is to understand two kinds of motivation. About 20% of people are motivated primarily by "toward" thinking and about 20% by "away from" thinking (with the other 60% falling between the two extremes). For example, a person who has an annual physical to avoid the pain and hardship of illness and disease is using an "away from" motivation. On the other hand, a person who has an annual physical to stay healthy and enjoy life is using "toward" motivation.

It's important to note, also, that motivations can change over time. For example, we may be motivated away from the feelings of ill health and lethargy and begin dieting and exercising. As we lose weight and feel better, we may unconsciously switch our motivation toward feeling more energetic and vibrant.

Neither motivation is better than the other and neither is right or wrong Recognizing which of these motivation types you are may make motivating yourself easier as you search for reasons to improve your lifestyle and health.

Getting Help in Taking Responsibility for Your Health

Being responsible for your health doesn't mean trying to go it alone. There are some fantastic physicians practicing today, and finding one with whom you can connect is a wonderful way to dig deeper and learn more about optimizing your health. This requires, however, that you take the time to learn and understand your unique situation and define your personal goals for improved health. This book is intended to help you do exactly that.

The opposite side of the coin is that you don't have to be satisfied with a patient/physician relationship that isn't fulfilling your needs. Don't be afraid to look for a physician who shares your passion for prevention and attacking problems at the root cause and not just focusing on treating symptoms.

It's All Connected

For me, one of the most interesting aspects in defining a preventive lifestyle is seeing how interconnected the systems in our bodies are. We talk about things like weight, heart disease, dental health, digestion, and thyroid health as if they're isolated factors, when in fact they're interconnected. Researchers understand this more each day. If you want to adopt a healthy lifestyle, you need to begin understanding these connections now. Even though this book is divided into separate topics, the interconnected nature of these systems will become clear.

Part 1: The Major Players

1

Coronary Artery Disease

Important idea #1: If your heart fails you, it really doesn't matter how healthy you are in other regards.

Even though the atrial fibrillation that took me to the ER turned out to be of little further concern, my ER visit turned out to have significant implications for my health. Not because of what I learned there, but because the entire experience opened my eyes to the importance of living a better lifestyle and pursuing optimum health, especially cardiac health.

Before we talk about assessing cardiac risk, let's talk about what coronary artery disease is.

Plaque = Coronary Artery Disease

We hear terms like heart disease and coronary artery disease and we know that doing certain things, like smoking, eating the wrong foods, and not exercising cause them. But what is coronary artery disease really?[1]

1. If you already have symptomatic heart disease, this book is not designed to take the place of a physician's care. The information here can certainly help your health and understanding, but you should be under the care of a cardiologist, preferably one who is happy that you've read a book like this and is pleased that you have become interested in preventive health.

For the purpose of our discussion, coronary artery disease is very simply *the presence of plaque within the coronary arteries.*

A very small amount of plaque may mean that you have a very slight case of coronary artery disease and plaque that has formed in such a way as to not cause an obstruction can be called non-obstructive plaque, but the presence of any plaque in your coronary arteries warrants concern.

Very simply, if you have plaque in your coronary arteries, you have coronary artery disease. Period.

That's the bad news.

The good news is that there are many ways in which you can help the situation.

- You can slow the rate at which plaque forms in your coronary arteries.
- You can stabilize the plaque so that it is much less likely to rupture.
- If you're lucky and you work very hard, you can possibly even reduce the amount of plaque in your coronary arteries, a feat that many cardiologists, however, believe is impossible.

Note: Even though a number of diseases can affect the heart, to keep from becoming cumbersome, I'll use the term *heart disease* generically to mean *coronary artery disease.*

It's important that we don't get hung up on plaque that obstructs versus plaque that doesn't obstruct. You'll learn later why all plaque, whether obstructive or not, poses a risk.

Traditional Testing for Heart Disease

Imagine having the following conversation with your child's teacher:

You: *How is my daughter doing in school this semester? Is she learning the required material?*

Teacher: *Based upon her age, and what we infer her socioeconomic status to be, as well as her assertions that she does homework on a* *regular basis, we believe she has a very high likelihood of having mastered this semester's materials acceptably.*

You: *Excuse me? What does this mean? Have you tested her on the material?*

Teacher: *No, we compared her socioeconomic status, apparent nutritional health, and her testimony that she does her homework regularly to a statistical model we have and there's a strong correlation between your daughter's parameters and students who mastered the coursework. Oh, and we measured the callouses on her writing fingers and they indicate that she's likely doing quite a bit of writing, which our statistical model shows increases by 22% her chances of having mastered the material. Overall, we feel very confident that she has mastered this semester's material.*

You: *I don't understand why you're comparing her to a statistical model instead of testing her. Do you ever plan on testing her?*

Teacher: *Only if she shows clear signs of having failed to master the material would we test her. As long as her parameters correlate acceptably to the statistical models of a successful population, we will assume that she is mastering the material.*

Does this sound like a school you would like your child to attend? Does estimating your child's performance by comparing indirect parameters to a statistical model sound like an ideal way to gauge her mastery of the subject matter? It certainly doesn't to me.

Yet this is how our medical culture typically measures the risk of coronary artery disease during routine preventive exams.

The Annual Exam

During your annual physical, your doctor will perform a variety of tests. The most common cardiac-related tests are the cholesterol test and blood pressure reading. Your physician uses these, in conjunction with your family history and body mass index (BMI) to measure your risk of cardiac disease. Note that I didn't say that the physician checks for heart disease—instead he or she measures your risk factors and compares them to a statistical model and, in the case of a stress test, tests you for the symptoms of coronary artery disease.

Note: A number of factors discussed here are influenced by gender but for the most part, I'll be gender-neutral.

What Are Risk Factors?

Risk factors are statistical models created by looking at a large group of people, measuring certain information (such as BMI,[1] cholesterol, or blood pressure) over a period of time, and comparing this information to the rate at which the individuals suffer a specific outcome, like heart attacks and heart-attack-related deaths. By comparing specific physiological markers such as obesity and blood pressure to the outcomes of an observed group, these observational studies provide risk factors for your doctor to use in gauging your risk of developing heart disease.

These sorts of observational studies can provide valuable clues as to what causes certain diseases within a population. For example, if the observational study shows the members of the group who were obese had a significantly greater chance of suffering a heart attack, the researchers would report this. Similarly, if the observational study showed those with elevated blood pressure were more likely to suffer a heart attack, the study would report this.

On the surface, this sounds like a reasonable and cost-effective way to assess individual risk and define clinical guidelines. Two problems arise, however, in trying to use observational studies as models for defining risk factors.

Mistaking Cause and Effect

The first problem is this: Using statistical models for defining risk factors creates errors when the researchers draw conclusions from what they see happening in the data.

For example, suppose the observational study showed that the obese members of the group had a 50% greater chance of having a heart attack than the individuals who were not obese. Then what?

---

1. The Body Mass Index (BMI) is defined as a person's body weight divided by the square of his or her height and is just a way of measuring how large a person is. Unfortunately, BMI has significant flaws, especially used as a risk factor. It ignores body composition (i.e., how much fat a person has) and automatically assumes that large people are large because they're fat, not because they're muscular. The nature of the BMI formula also means that a short person with the same body fat percentage as a tall person is more likely to be labeled "obese."

Researchers would likely report that there's a correlation between obesity and heart attack risk.

What does "correlation" mean in a case like this? It means that when one value (e.g., the person's body mass index) changes, the other factor (e.g., heart attack rate) changes in a predictable proportion.

I can make up a correlation graph of that relationship:

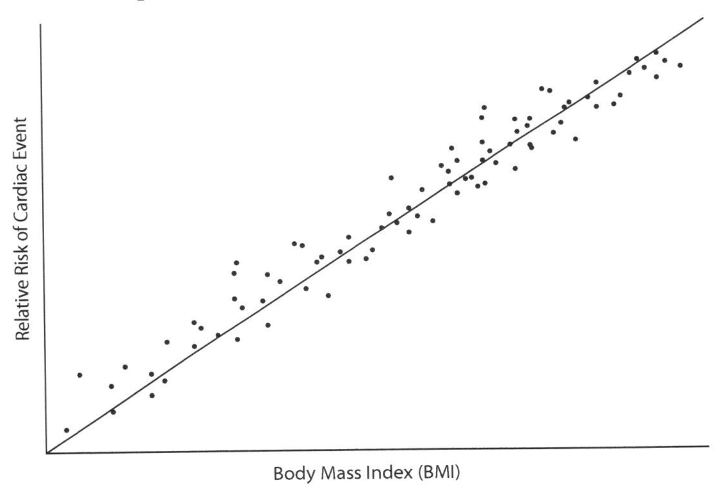

One possible conclusion from this fictitious example is that obesity causes heart disease. But that's not necessarily true just because they're correlated. It only means that they are correlated and correlation does not necessarily prove causation. At best it means that the relationship warrants further investigation.

The significance of this distinction is clear in the next example.

According to a 2007 study by the Center for Disease Control (CDC), 57% of the people who died in the United States died in a hospital. There is, therefore, a stronger correlation between death and being in a hospital than being anywhere else. Would it be correct to say that going to a hospital is the greatest cause of death in this country? Of course not. Drawing a conclusion like that would require overlooking the fact that the very same things that bring people to a hospital (illness and injury) are the things that cause death. Being in the hospital and dying are not causally linked; they just both result from the same thing: the illness and injury that brought the person to the hospital in the first place.

Returning to the obesity versus heart disease correlation, does this correlation allow us to conclude with certainty that obesity causes heart disease? A better question asks: does that conclusion overlook a common cause of both obesity and heart disease?

In fact, being obese does not cause heart disease. Instead, heart disease and obesity share a very significant cause: high glucose and insulin levels produced by becoming insulin-resistant.

Overlooking the role of insulin resistance, with its companions elevated glucose and insulin levels, and drawing the wrong conclusion that obesity causes heart disease leads practitioners to focus on a symptom of the same disease instead of focusing on the disease. Stated another way, telling obese people to lose weight in order to reduce their risk of heart disease is attacking a symptom (obesity) instead of attacking the cause (elevated glucose and insulin). The typical result is a failed attempt at weight loss and an increased rate of heart disease as both physician and patient overlook the damaging effects of insulin resistance.

Individuals Behave Differently Than Population Groups Do

One example of a population study that's used to define individual risk is the hemoglobin A1C test. The A1C test uses a mathematical model, derived from sampling hundreds of people, to estimate from a single blood test what your blood glucose level has been over the past 100 days. The A1C is a useful test in several circumstances, but there's enough imprecision in the mathematical model that your average glucose level can vary significantly from what the model estimates it to have been.

One of the most commonly used formulas for converting an A1C value to an average blood glucose level states that there can be as much as a 50-point range in the calculated blood glucose levels. In many patients, this variance is wide enough to make the difference between reporting harmful historical blood glucose levels and reporting harmless ones. While estimating one's past glucose levels with an A1C calculation is better than having no data at all, assuming that every individual's glucose levels precisely match the population group can lead to significantly inaccurate picture of the individual's glucose history.

Statistical Models Can Be Useful

Don't get me wrong. I'm not saying that statistical models and observational studies are useless. They can be an effective tool for helping to identify areas for further research, perhaps with a clinical trial, and for setting public guidelines (for example, "smoking increases your risk of lung cancer and heart disease"). They can also be useful when there's no other way to paint a picture of what's been happening (e.g., the A1C's estimate of a person's blood glucose history).

As useful as they can be, however, statistical models do not determine if a *specific individual* has a *specific disease*, in this case, in determining whether or not an individual has coronary artery disease.

Some Specific Problems with the Risk Factors in Use Today

Blood Pressure

High blood pressure is quite damaging to the body, producing cracks and fissures in arterial walls. As you'll learn later, these cracks and fissures become breeding grounds for the formation of cardiac plaque. High blood pressure also damages the heart itself, the kidneys, and the brain. There's no doubt about it—high blood pressure is a significant contributor to ill health and the presence of high blood pressure is a strong indicator that a person is at much higher risk for heart disease.

But while it's prudent to view high blood pressure as a significant risk factor for heart disease, it doesn't work in reverse: Normal blood pressure doesn't mean you're immune from heart disease.

At the risk of getting off topic, I believe there's a tendency to view high blood pressure as a disease in itself, compelling doctor and patient to attack the condition with medications to lower blood pressure rather than attack the root cause of high blood pressure, which is often systemic inflammation that causes arteries to become rigid and inflexible, frequently coupled with potassium and magnesium deficiencies. Attacking the sources of inflammation in the body can reduce blood pressure without needing to take a blood pressure medication for the rest of your life.

This is a place for a common sense approach because sometimes it's necessary to attack the symptom first and then attack the root cause. Here, a physician may start a patient on a blood pressure medication to lower the blood pressure and allow the body to begin healing. In parallel, the physician and patient should then investigate inflammatory causes and address them as well.[1]

Too often, however, patients and physicians become focused on the symptom and once the blood pressure medication brings results, all efforts at making lifestyle changes to deal with the inflammation are forgotten.

Your physician's job is to help you quickly minimize or prevent further damage to your body and, yes, blood pressure medication does that. But the deeper question is this: Do you want to be someone who is content to treat symptoms, perhaps taking medication your whole life, or do you want to correct problems at the source?

Cholesterol

There are so many misconceptions about cholesterol and its role in cardiac health that cholesterol gets its own chapter. For now, suffice it to say that simply stating high cholesterol causes coronary artery disease is wrong. It's not just about LDL and HDL either. See Chapter 2 for more information on the role that cholesterol plays in your life. You may be very surprised.

Fitness

How often do we read of cyclists, professional soccer players, marathoners, and countless others who are clearly quite physically fit yet who have collapsed and died of a heart attack? Running guru Jim Fixx, credited by many as having started the 1970s fitness craze, was clearly an exceptional example of physical fitness, yet he died of a heart attack when he was 52. The autopsy revealed that atherosclerosis had blocked one coronary artery 95%, a second at 85%, and a third at 70%.

---

1. According to Dr. Michael Eades, author of *The Protein Power Lifeplan*, most Americans are deficient in magnesium and potassium. I talk more about this in Appendix I.

Again, don't get me wrong. I'm not saying that exercise is bad (though there are some misconceptions about aerobic exercise, as I discuss later). I am saying that it's clear that being fit does not mean that a person is therefore free of coronary artery disease. Do you cycle on a regular basis? Do you run? Swim? Jog? Great. You may be very fit, indeed. But being fit doesn't take the place of accurately assessing yourself for coronary artery disease. Nor does a stress test. Read on.

The False Reassurance of the Stress Test

Approximately 5 to 10 million cardiac stress tests are performed every year and they are currently an integral part of assessing cardiac health.

It could be argued that a stress test is far more useful than comparing cholesterol or blood pressure to a statistical model because a stress test shows exactly how an individual's heart performs under stress. And indeed a stress test is a useful tool in measuring certain aspects of cardiac health. However, it is not useful as a routine test for measuring the presence of coronary artery disease. This is because a stress test doesn't rule out the presence of coronary artery disease; passing a stress test only shows that there's not enough coronary artery disease present to show up on a stress test.

It's true that sufficiently advanced coronary artery disease will eventually impair cardiac function sufficiently to show up on a stress test. What's unfortunate, however, is that the body's ability to adapt to the disease's slow progression (by enlarging other coronary arteries, for example) typically means that by the time coronary artery disease shows up on a stress test, the person's heart has suffered enough impairment that intervention is much more likely to be required.

According to cardiologist William Davis, "Stress tests usually detect blockages when they meet or exceed 70%—anything less than this is not detected. A person with dozens of lesser blockages of, say, 20%, 30%, 40%, or 50% will therefore not be detected by stress tests."[1] I don't know about you, but I'd much rather find out about my coronary artery disease decades before I collapse on a treadmill and find that I'm facing a stent or bypass surgery.

How Should I Determine Whether I Have Coronary Artery Disease?

How do doctors test for glaucoma? They use a wand or a puff of air to directly measure the pressure within the eyeball. How does a doctor determine someone has cervical cancer? By swabbing some cells and examining them under a microscope. How does a doctor determine if you have a broken bone? By x-raying the bone and checking for a break. Do you see a pattern here?

Recall our definition of coronary artery disease: coronary artery disease is the presence of plaque in your coronary arteries. So, how do you test for coronary artery disease? *If you want to know if you have coronary artery disease, you check your coronary arteries to see if they contain any plaque.* Simple, isn't it?

For some baffling reason, though, this eludes many people, including many physicians.

The Coronary Calcium Scan

You probably already know what a CT (computed tomography) scan is. You may have already had one. A CT scanner is a sophisticated combination of x-ray machine and imaging computer that can produce 3-D images of almost any part of your body. Doctors can use this same CT scanner to take very fast pictures of your coronary arteries and see if plaque is present.

---

1. Dr. William Davis is a prevention cardiologist in Milwaukee, WI. He is also the founder of the Track Your Plaque program for preventing and reversing heart disease. He is the author of *Track Your Plaque*, a book on prevention cardiology, and *Wheat Belly*, an in-depth look at the harmful effects of today's wheat on human health.

A coronary calcium scan is safe, inexpensive, and very accurate. How inexpensive? I've found cardiologists in my area who perform the scan and interpret the results for $49.

Yes, $49.

Then why don't we routinely test every adult for the presence of coronary artery plaque?

The answer lies in a mixture of human nature, economics, and ignorance.

- Many patients and physicians don't know about the coronary calcium scan.
- Many physicians, and some patients, do know about a coronary calcium scan but they've been confused by inaccurate reporting that mistakes this test for a more expensive test called a *CT angiogram* that involves injecting a contrast medium and exposing the patient to a much larger amount of radiation.
- Many physicians believe that there's nothing a person can do about coronary artery plaque that's already there, so as long as a patient has no symptoms (or a patient passes a stress test), the presence of plaque needn't be directly addressed.
- Astonishingly, insurance companies very rarely cover the minimal cost of a coronary calcium scan. I suspect that is because many insurance companies do not believe that patients will be compelled by the results of a coronary calcium scan to make lifestyle changes. Moreover, even if patients do make lifestyle changes, they'll probably be insured by a different insurance company twenty years in the future when the cost-savings of those lifestyle changes are fully realized.

How Does a Coronary Calcium Scan Work?

Coronary plaque contains a mixture of substances, including white blood cells, cholesterol, and calcium. Plaque has a lifecycle and can exist in a dynamic state, starting as soft plaque (with little or no embedded calcium); after a year or two, it becomes calcified.

Because a CT scanner is very good at identifying the presence of calcium, CT scan technology lends itself well to quickly and easily identifying the presence of coronary plaque in your arteries, without any contrast medium, catheterization, or other intervention. The CT scanner is so fast that the images are taken between the beats of your heart. What's more, cadaver studies have shown that calcium is present in a rather consistent amount: 20% of coronary plaque is calcium. This fact allows the CT scan to *quantify* the amount of coronary plaque, as you'll soon read.

Best of all, because the amount of radiation from a coronary calcium scan is so low, it's reasonable to repeat the calcium scan periodically to continue assessing your plaque burden.[1]

The Calcium Scan Report

Because the calcium scan uses the presence of calcium to determine the presence of plaque, the results are reported numerically, as a total volume of plaque present in the arteries. For example, a score of 225 means that a person's coronary arteries contain 225 cubic millimeters of plaque.

Think about how the usefulness of this number compares to the much less defined risk assessment that a traditional annual physical entails. Which of these series of events sounds more like effective preventive medicine to you?

Monitoring Your Cardiac Health — Method 1: The current method

Your cholesterol, blood pressure, and BMI are recorded and used to determine your risk against statistical models. Your tests show a relatively low risk of heart disease, so you are reassured that you're living a healthy enough lifestyle.

After years of being reassured by your favorable comparison to risk models, one day you have a more comprehensive physical that includes a stress test (or perhaps you were compelled to have a stress test because you felt dizzy or light-headed while

---

1. A standard chest x-ray exposes you to 0.15 mSv, a relatively minor amount of radiation; a coronary calcium scan for tracking cardiac plaque exposes you to 0.4–0.6 mSv if performed on an EBT (Electron Beam Tomography) device and 0.6–2.0 mSv if performed on a 64-slice CT device. Nakazato 2009; Stolzmann 2009, cited by William Davis in *Track Your Plaque.*

exercising or climbing stairs). Amazingly, the stress test shows that one or more of your coronary arteries is 80% blocked.

That afternoon you're in the cardiac catheterization lab getting a stent inserted, with all of its risks and complications. (**Note**: This is the most desirable way this sort of thing can turn out. Many times the first sign of advanced coronary artery disease is a fatal heart attack.)

Monitoring Your Cardiac Health — Method 2: An improved method

In addition to the routine blood work every year, now that you're 43, your doctor sends you for a coronary calcium scan that costs half as much as a pair of running shoes. The result from this safe, painless, completely non-invasive test is not good: It shows that you have 100 cubic millimeters of coronary plaque, an amount that's worse than 90% of the other 43-year-olds out there.

Knowing for certain that this plaque is present, you and your doctor implement a set of lifestyle changes (like the ones discussed later in this book) to both prevent more plaque and to reduce what you have already. Repeating the scan periodically allows you and your physician to monitor the success of your lifestyle changes and alter them accordingly.

It's pretty clear to me how I'd like to find out about my coronary artery disease. However, many doctors push patients toward Method 1 with all of its uncertainty and they are less enthusiastic about proactively measuring coronary calcium in their adult patients. To illustrate the pervasiveness of this attitude, let's compare attitudes toward mammograms with attitudes toward coronary calcium scanning.

Mammograms versus Coronary Calcium Scanning

As with coronary artery disease, a variety of risk factors influence your chance of developing breast cancer. Most notable is gender: women have 100 times the risk of developing breast cancer as men.[1] Increased age and certain genetic factors, like BRCA1 and BRCA2 gene mutations, also increase the risk of breast cancer. As with coronary artery disease, family history, body weight, and

1. Risk factors obtained from National Cancer Institute informational publications.

physical activity level are also factors in assessing breast cancer risk.

Despite these various factors that increase a woman's risk of breast cancer, traditional medical thinking doesn't soften their recommendations for mammograms based upon risk factors (other than gender, that is). The National Cancer Institute (NCI) unilaterally recommends that *every woman over the age of 40 have a mammogram every 12 to 24 months*. When the NCI does bring risk factors into the picture, they do so to strengthen the recommendations ever further, advising women in higher-risk categories to weigh the benefits of starting routine mammograms prior to age 40.

In sharp contrast to advice on mammograms, many physicians will not recommend coronary calcium scans to patients unless the patient *is already at high risk* for heart disease. This doesn't seem like sound advice to me when I consider the words of prevention cardiologist Dr. William Davis, "The practical reality is that 90% of future heart attacks will not be predicted by any of the conventional tests, a 9 out of 10 chance that the battery of testing you just submitted to *will have failed to identify an impending heart attack*."[1]

Many physicians, and medical publications, warn consumers away from calcium scanning due to concerns about radiation, often confusing calcium scanning with the higher radiation contrast angiography. Yet these concerns about radiation exposure are not considered prohibiting for mammograms. In fact, the NCI advises that "the risk of harm from this radiation exposure is low, but repeated x-rays have the potential to cause cancer. The benefits, however, nearly always outweigh the risk."

All in all, the recommendations given to women regarding mammograms seem logical and beneficial whereas the dramatic difference in attitude toward coronary calcium scanning is baffling. It's not a stretch at all to say that many patients are advised not to have a coronary calcium scan unless they first prove themselves worthy of greater scrutiny by repeatedly failing a cholesterol test or showing abnormalities on a stress test. It's unfathomable to me that a doctor would dissuade or even be noncommittal about calcium scans ("I can't recommend it, but have one if you want," a

---

1. Track Your Plaque.

friend's physician told him) when they will recommend that every woman over the age of 40 have a mammogram.

Repeating the Calcium Scan

Once you've decided to have a coronary calcium scan, how often should you repeat the test?

That depends on a variety of factors, not the least of which is your age and your previous scores. If, for example, you have a calcium scan at 40 and it shows a plaque burden that places you in the 99 percentile of plaque (i.e., you have more cardiac plaque than 99% of those of your age and gender), then you'll probably want to keep a close eye on your plaque and repeat the scan in 12–24 months. A 40-year-old person with a zero calcium score, on the other hand, may be fine waiting five years for the next scan. The most important thing is that the coronary calcium scan is an effective tool for objectively measuring cardiac plaque, far superior to statistical models for measuring your individual risk. Planning the strategy for monitoring your calcium scan is a great topic of discussion for you and your physician, providing your physician is open-minded enough to appreciate the scan.

Studies have shown that coronary plaque can grow at a rate of 30% per year, doubling in amount every three years. Thus, a calcium score of 100 today can become 1,000 in about a decade.

The obvious question is why do we not skip all the testing and just implement heart-healthy lifestyle changes as a precaution and not worry about the coronary calcium scan? The best answer is probably "human nature." Considering how few people are willing to make lifestyle changes in the face of certain risk, I imagine far fewer would be compelled to make changes in response to an unsubstantiated one. Plus, with a numerical measurement of your coronary plaque, it will be possible to measure your success in combating its growth.

Coronary calcium scans were originally done using EBT (electron beam tomography), which provides a more accurate scan with even less radiation. Unfortunately, CT scanners are replacing most EBT scanners today for a variety of reasons. See Appendix O for more comparison between these two technologies.

The Risks of Coronary Artery Plaque

We've talked a great deal about coronary artery disease and the fact that having plaque in your coronary arteries signals coronary artery disease, but what exactly are the risks of having plaque? We already know the answer or at least we think we do: Plaque builds up and clogs our arteries, which causes obstructions. When the obstruction has completely blocked an artery, we have a heart attack.

Unfortunately, that's the problem with simple explanations: they're often incorrect. As H. L. Mencken stated, "For every complex problem, there is an answer that is clear, simple, and wrong."

Obstructive versus Non-Obstructive Plaque

When we hear about coronary artery disease, we typically hear about blockages, also called obstructions. We hear that an artery is 50% blocked or that we have 90% blockages in three coronary arteries and need emergency bypass surgery. We hear about angioplasty (balloon surgery) that can open clogged arteries and about stents that widen occluded arterial passages.

All of this may lead us to think that the danger of arterial plaque is the slowly forming obstructive plaque that gradually makes the arterial passage smaller and smaller until it finally closes up. While this is one possible way that heart attacks occur, it may surprise you that fewer than 30% of heart attacks happen in this way.

So, if obstructive plaque represents fewer than 30% heart attack risks, what causes the other 70%? Non-obstructive plaque, plaque that occludes less than 50% of a coronary artery and therefore will not show up on a stress test.

How can non-obstructive plaque cause a heart attack if it doesn't obstruct?

That question is answered more fully later. For now, just imagine a crusty, brittle segment of arterial wall, constantly being flexed and pounded from elevated blood pressure until a piece of the scab breaks away. The site of this plaque rupture quickly forms a blood clot, which causes a heart attack. Because of this, the fast-forming clot from ruptured, *non-obstructive* plaque poses an often-overlooked risk while we focus primarily on obstructions.

All Plaque Is Evil

As will become increasingly clear, even though obstructive and non-obstructive plaque cause heart attacks in different ways, all plaque is evil and needs to be rendered inactive as rapidly as possible.

If non-obstructive plaque causes more heart attacks than obstructive plaque, why do we hear so much about obstructive plaque and so little about non-obstructive plaque? It's probably because today's medical care is much better at detecting and treating blockages than at treating non-obstructive plaque. In fact, many physicians believe that once non-obstructive plaque is present, there's nothing a person can do to reduce the threat of a heart attack from it.

However, I share the optimism displayed by a number of forward-thinking cardiologists, such as Dr. William Davis, who believe that it's very possible to inactivate cardiac plaque, thus greatly reducing the risk of plaque rupture. The same strategies that inactivate plaque will also slow, or even stop, the formation of additional plaque, further reducing the risk of heart attack. Reports from patients who have achieved substantial reductions in their rate of plaque growth and even reduced the amount of plaque they have add credibility to this belief.

The Most Important Points from This Chapter

- Most routine physical exams assess the health of a patient's coronary arteries by indirect means, using indicators and risk factors.
- A typical stress test doesn't reveal the presence of coronary plaque unless 70% or more of the artery is blocked.
- Slowly forming arterial blockages do not cause most heart attacks; they're just historically the most treatable kind of plaque, so that's what we hear about the most.
- Most heart attacks are caused when non-obstructive plaque ruptures.

- The best way to gauge the presence of coronary artery disease is by using an inexpensive coronary calcium scan to directly measure the amount of plaque you have in your coronary arteries.
- A great deal of misinformation surrounds the coronary calcium scan, with many people mistaking it for CT contrast angiography.
- Despite what many cardiologists think, we can reduce the risk of plaque rupture and in some cases, reduce the amount of coronary plaque we have.

If You Want to Take Action Immediately

- Have a coronary calcium scan so that you know how much plaque you have in your coronary arteries.
- Share the results with your physician.

  This vital test turns the abstract (your *risk* of heart disease based upon *indicators*) into the tangible (do *you* have plaque in *your* coronary arteries *right now*?).

2

Fat Is Where It's At

The subject of fat and cholesterol as they relate to optimal health is a hotly debated subject in nutrition and health. There are those who argue that fat should be the primary component in our diet, those who argue just as strongly for avoiding fat as much as possible, and those who advocate every imaginable position in-between.

I want to repeat again the importance of recognizing that we're all different and things that are best for one person (or what a scientific study shows is best for a group of people) cannot be guaranteed to work best for you or me. I cannot repeat this enough: Whatever you read or whatever anyone (even a physician) tells you about an optimal diet, only proper testing can reveal whether a particular diet is ideal for you. No scientific study on a group of people can tell you with certainty what is optimal for you.

In my research, I have identified a number of oversimplifications, dangerous generalities, and important guidelines for you to keep in mind as you investigate what works best for you.

What Is Cholesterol?

Cholesterol is a sterol, a type of organic molecule. Sterols occur in virtually every plant and animal life form, with cholesterol being the most common sterol in mammals.

Cholesterol plays a variety of crucial roles in the body. It is a starting material for an array of steroids that are vital to the body, including vitamin D, testosterone, and estrogen. Found in nearly every cell of the body, cholesterol is a principal component of cell membranes, giving the cell membrane its necessary strength and flexibility and allowing the cell to very effectively limit what materials can enter and exit the cell.

Volumes have been written about the importance of cholesterol in the body but suffice it to say that cholesterol is an absolutely vital component of the body that is present in nearly every cell. Insufficient cholesterol causes cancer, dementia, and an array of hormonal problems.

Is Cholesterol Friend or Foe?

A *Time* magazine cover in 1984 showed a frowning face made out of bacon and eggs and the article inside delivering the bad news: Cholesterol causes heart disease. This cover elevated the public's awareness of cholesterol and its perceived dangers.

The following decades brought an onslaught of warnings about eating foods containing cholesterol and about the benefits of low-fat foods. Margarine and corn oil displaced butter and lard. It wasn't long before *low-fat* became synonymous with *healthy*. In fact, the "low-fat is good/cholesterol is bad" message has become so thoroughly entrenched that many people believe that for optimum health we need as little cholesterol as possible in our body. One misguided person posted on a health and fitness forum that even though she had been eating very well and exercising regularly, she "couldn't understand why her cholesterol level wasn't zero by now." She should be glad that her cholesterol level hasn't reached zero because if it had, she'd probably be dead!

Such thinking illustrates perfectly how people have come to misunderstand cholesterol and its role. Even people who understand that there's a "good" cholesterol called HDL and a "bad" cholesterol called LDL are still decades behind the research in their thinking and are embracing a dangerously oversimplified model.

Types of Cholesterol in the Body

You may have heard of HDL (high-density lipoprotein) and LDL (low-density lipoprotein) and maybe even you're familiar with the term VLDL (very low-density lipoprotein). Clearly there's more to the cholesterol issue than what we refer to as *cholesterol*. How many types of cholesterol do you think there are in the body? Just these three? Five? Ten? Twenty?

It's a trick question: there's only one type of cholesterol in the body. Cholesterol is cholesterol is cholesterol.

Then why do we hear so much about "types of cholesterol" and "good" cholesterol and "bad" cholesterol? The answer to that hinges on the nature of cholesterol itself, a fatty, oily substance. As we learned in elementary school, oil and water do not mix. This means that without some way of overcoming the incompatibility of oil and water, cholesterol could never be transported effectively in the bloodstream without clumping and separating.

The body overcomes this challenge by enclosing cholesterol in a special container, called a phospholipid ("phospho" comes from "phosphate," which is part of the container, and "lipid" meaning fat). The outer surface of this phospholipid shell has chemical properties that allow it to disperse and travel effectively within the watery bloodstream, carrying the cholesterol to the countless destinations where it can perform its vital functions.

These lipid transport containers, sometimes referred to simply as "lipids," come in many different forms, even though they all carry cholesterol. These different forms of lipid transport vehicles are what many people mistake for different types of cholesterol when, in fact, they're just different vehicles, all carrying the same passenger.

As we'll see later, these different forms of lipid particles (cholesterol transport vehicles) are the key to understanding how cardiac plaque forms and why merely concerning ourselves with cholesterol levels (or even just LDL and HDL levels) is outdated and can even be dangerously simplistic.

Key Members of the Phospholipid Family

HDL — Regarded as the "good" cholesterol, HDL's primary role is to gather up used cholesterol and transport it to be removed from the body or recycled into new cholesterol.

LDL — Regarded as the "bad" cholesterol, LDL's primary role is to distribute newly created cholesterol throughout the body, depositing it in the many locations where it's needed.

Triglycerides — Triglycerides are a group of three fatty acids and a glycerol molecule. While they are a very necessary energy source, high triglyceride levels contribute to coronary plaque formation and excessively high levels can cause other complications in the body, including unfavorable lipid particles, pancreatitis, and fatty liver. As you'll learn later, sugar (in fact, most any carbohydrate), not fats, is the most common cause of elevated triglycerides.

Very early into research about cholesterol and health, I became skeptical that LDL is as harmful as claimed.

If cholesterol is so vital that virtually every cell in the body is capable of making cholesterol if it needs to, then why is the lipid particle responsible for distributing this vital component labeled "bad" cholesterol?

And why is taking cholesterol where it needs to go considered bad?

It seemed to me then, and I believe it even more strongly now, that unilaterally labeling LDL as "bad" is dangerously oversimplified.

Sources of Cholesterol

Where does the cholesterol in our body come from? That's easy, right? It comes from the animal products we eat, like red meat, eggs, and cheese. I've heard that, too, but it's wrong.

It's true that many of the foods we eat contain some cholesterol, but the cholesterol we eat accounts for only about 20% of the cholesterol in our bodies. The other 80% is manufactured by our bodies, primarily by our liver. Cholesterol is so important to the body, however, that the body manufactures approximately three grams of cholesterol per day, which is ten times the recommended dietary intake of cholesterol. This means that for most people, no matter how much cholesterol we eat, it will make very little difference in the cholesterol levels in our bloodstream.

This brings two obvious questions: If the cholesterol we eat has very little to do with the cholesterol that results in our bloodstream and our body makes most of the cholesterol we need, why do some people have abnormally high cholesterol and why might our cholesterol level change over time? The very simple answer is diet and genetics.

But wait! I just said that the cholesterol we eat doesn't affect the amount of cholesterol in our bloodstream and now I'm saying that diet affects the amount of cholesterol in our bloodstream. How can both statements be true?

Here's why: The cholesterol you eat trivially affects the cholesterol in your bloodstream; however, the other foods you eat significantly affect your liver and its production of cholesterol, most importantly, the type of lipid particles that your liver produces.

Current Theories of Cholesterol Health

To put this information in the proper context, it will be helpful to know something about current theories on cholesterol health. After all, much of the advice that's offered by food manufacturers, drug companies, and healthcare professionals is borne out of the current theories on cholesterol as they pertain to heart disease. Understanding these theories, including their strengths and weaknesses, will help you determine which of today's health advice is worthwhile.

The mainstream theories on cholesterol health condense into two fundamental arguments:

- Eating cholesterol (and saturated fats in general) causes heart disease.
  (This is called the *diet-health theory.*)
- High cholesterol levels in the bloodstream cause heart disease.
  (This is called the *lipid hypothesis.*)

Unfortunately, these theories are full of holes. The many flaws of the diet-heath theory include data manipulation (in studying diets and disease from different countries, the researchers purposely excluded data from those countries that didn't prove their theory), incorrect cause of death (as many as half of the deaths attributed to cardiac disease were caused by something else), and dubious data on the amount of saturated fat intake. The net result is that blaming saturated fat intake for heart disease is baseless, with numerous, far more credible studies being released in recent years that show saturated fats to be beneficial at best and benign at worst.

The second prevailing cholesterol theory, the lipid hypothesis, doesn't address diet. It merely says that elevated cholesterol levels cause heart disease. This theory, too, has been debunked by numerous worldwide studies that show no difference in cholesterol levels between those who have heart disease and those who do not. In fact, many studies show that those with excessively low cholesterol levels have increased risk of heart disease, cancer, and dementia.

The implication from these two theories is that eating fats elevates your cholesterol level, which clogs your arteries. It didn't matter that the message from these flawed theories was, as a result, also deeply flawed. All it took for this way of thinking to become entrenched was the backing of politicians eager to make a name for themselves and pharmaceutical companies eager to make a profit by selling medications that lower cholesterol in the blood.[1] The net result is today's commonly held belief that eating fat clogs our arteries and causes heart disease.

---

1. See Appendix A.

The Kernels of Truth in the Diet-Health Theory

It's obvious to me that the diet-health theory is inaccurate. Study after study shows that simply eating fat does not cause heart disease. In fact, low-fat diets can increase the risk of heart disease [1] and diabetes.[2]

However, I've come to realize that the human body is so complex that rarely can we make broad statements claiming something to always be harmful or harmless. Such is the case with saturated fats. Despite all the evidence disputing the link between saturated fat intake and heart disease, there are some very relevant kernels of truth that eating certain types of fats contributes to heart disease. Examining these specific risks associated with saturated fat intake may provide a clue as to why some studies show saturated fats to be a heart disease promoter while some show saturated fats to be benign or beneficial.

Oxidized Cholesterol

Cholesterol has been a principal component of the human diet since the beginning of recorded history. I contend that human genetics has not changed sufficiently in the past 50 years or so to cause heart disease to become the rampant killer that it is today.

One significant difference between our distant ancestors' consumption of cholesterol and ours, however, is oxidation. When our ancestors ate animal products, they didn't subject them to the harsh processing and cooking methods that we employ today. These processes cause the cholesterol in our food to become heavily oxidized, which turns beneficial cholesterol into something very different.

---

1. Countless studies cited by Taubes and others show increased heart disease with low-fat diets. An early study that caught my attention is by G Cristakis, Effect of the anti-coronary club program on coronary heart disease risk-factor status. *Journal of the American Medical Association* 1966;198:(6):129–135. It's not difficult to find many other studies saying the same thing.

2. Low-fat diets invariably replace fat calories with carbohydrates (typically whole grains). The resultant elevated glucose and insulin levels pave the way for Type 2 diabetes (and in the case of the increasingly common wheat gluten sensitivities, many say Type 1 diabetes, as well).

Advanced Glycated End Products (AGEs)

Glycation is a biochemical term for something you're probably familiar with: caramelization. Caramelizing something requires that you bond it to sugar, producing a gooey substance that sticks to nearly anything. This is essentially what happens in the body in the presence of high levels of blood glucose: saturated fats bond to sugar (glucose) in the body, producing highly reactive, damaging compounds called Advanced Glycated End Products (AGEs). See Chapter 6 for more about AGEs.

Dyslipidemia

Unlike oxidation and glycation, which are things that we do to the saturated fats we eat, an additional risk from saturated fats is intrinsic to the saturated fats themselves: They require a bit more work for the body to break down into healthy lipid particles. When we cannot effectively metabolize saturated fats into healthy lipid particles, we typically produce higher levels of unfavorable particles, those causing heart disease. This disorder of lipid metabolism is called *dyslipidemia*.[1]

This inability to effectively metabolize saturated fats seems to be a factor, however, only when we are already suffering from impaired lipid metabolism, and it is typically not a problem when we are able to metabolize lipids effectively. This is nonetheless a critical point, as it is likely a significant factor in explaining why most people do well with diets that contain a significant amount of saturated fats while a small percentage of people do not. To me, the fact that a small percentage of people have dysfunctional lipid metabolism, which prevents them from effectively metabolizing saturated fats, is not an indictment on saturated fats. Rather, it points to the foods and lifestyle that caused their dysfunction in the first place, most likely their decades-long, glucose-inducing diet of sugars and grains, combined with unhealthy vegetable oils.

Later, I'll talk about measuring your postprandial triglyceride levels to determine if you are one of the rare people whose body is less effective at metabolizing saturated fats. Measuring only your

1. *Dyslipidemia* is sometimes used to mean the presence of elevated lipid levels, no matter their cause. In the context above, dyslipidemia specifically means the inability to effectively metabolize ingested lipids.

fasting triglycerides, which is the typical way our triglycerides are measured, will never tell you as clearly whether this is the case.

The Kernel of Truth in the Lipid Hypothesis

Despite my argument against the lipid hypothesis, you may be surprised to learn that our lipid profile does significantly influence our risk of heart disease. The problem with the lipid hypothesis, however, is that even though it's focused in the correct general direction (lipids), by looking at total cholesterol or even LDL, it is overlooking the real lipid-based factors that cause heart disease.

THE REAL CULPRITS IN THE LIPID SAGA

If the lipid hypothesis that LDL is bad and HDL is good is dangerously simplistic, then what accounts for the buildup of cardiac plaque? Is cholesterol, or are lipids, a factor at all?

Yes, lipids *are* a significant factor. The problem is that today's commonplace advice is lagging well behind the research. Before researchers discovered HDL and LDL, they knew only to look at total cholesterol in the body. For a while, the medical community talked only about the importance of maintaining a healthy cholesterol level in the blood. Having a cholesterol level above 200 or so, they said, was unhealthy. Before too long, however, when LDL and HDL were better understood, the lipid picture became a little clearer: LDL became known as "bad" cholesterol and HDL became known as "good" cholesterol, with physicians and pharmaceutical companies (and all who are influenced by them) lagging behind research and continuing to tell us to lower our LDL and increase our HDL for optimum health. Instead of focusing solely on LDL and HDL, however, we should be focusing on what's really the single most important factor in lipid health: *particles.*

Particles, Not Cholesterol

If you've ever seen a lab report showing your LDL cholesterol, you've probably noticed that your LDL level is listed as "LDL-C" (or your doctor may just call it "LDL"). The designation *LDL-C* means "LDL cholesterol" and is a measurement of the total amount of cholesterol that is carried by LDL particles in a given volume of blood. If you'll recall from earlier in the chapter, however, cholesterol doesn't float freely in the bloodstream. Because cholesterol is a fatty substance, it is contained in phospholipid particles that are designed to travel well in blood and carry the cholesterol safely to its destination. Measuring just the total LDL-cholesterol in a given volume of blood doesn't give the complete picture because it ignores the *number* of phospholipid particles that a specific individual is using to carry that LDL.

It's okay if this is a bit confusing. I'll illustrate with an analogy.

To understand the distinction between measuring total LDL versus measuring LDL particles, think about it in terms of traffic on a highway. Saying that one million people travel a given highway each day doesn't provide a very complete picture of how crowded the highway is. After all, *people* don't clog a highway, *vehicles* do. Stated another way, there's a very big difference between a million people traveling on a highway with only one person in each car versus the same million people per day if there are four or five people in each car. Measuring just the people (LDL-C) doesn't tell us nearly as much as counting the total number of cars (LDL particles, or *LDL-P*) on our hypothetical highway.

How does this car analogy translate to you and me? Imagine that you and I had the same LDL-C value reported on our most recent physical. Because the LDL-C value measures only the *amount* of cholesterol contained in LDL particles, this value tells us nothing about the *number* of LDL particles you have versus the number that I have. You and I could have the *same* LDL-C value and yet one of us could have *double* the number of LDL particles in our blood.

Why is this distinction important? *Because the number of LDL particles in your blood is far more relevant to your risk of heart disease than your total amount of LDL.*[1]

---

1. Otvos, JD, Mora, A, et al. Clinical implications of discordance between low-density lipoprotein cholesterol and particle number. *Journal of Clinical Lipidology* 2011; 5, 105–113.

   Snidermana, AD, et al. Triglycerides and small dense LDL: The twin Achilles heels of the Friedewald formula. *Clinical Biochemistry* 2003; 36 499–504.

   Brunzell, JD et al. lipoprotein management in patients with cardiometabolic risk. *Journal of the American College of Cardiology* 2008; 51:1512–1524.

In other words, if you compare the particle count (LDL-P) for two people, the person with a *higher* particle count is at higher risk for heart disease, *even if their LDL-C values are exactly the same.*

Think about this for a moment: Virtually every study that tries to relate LDL cholesterol to heart attack risk uses LDL-C, not LDL-P. Thus, these studies are lumping together those with *favorable* particle counts and those with *unfavorable* particle counts, just because they have similar LDL-C values.

This is quite likely the biggest reason why so many people with "normal LDL" have heart attacks and so many people with "high LDL" do not: because simply measuring the amount of LDL-C and ignoring the LDL-P (particle count) doesn't reveal how healthy or unhealthy a our lipids are.

Read the previous paragraph again. It's that important.

The bigger implication here is that continually attempting to drive our LDL-C ever lower and lower isn't attacking the problem of unfavorable lipid particles and, in fact, is probably harmful, as excessively lowered levels of LDL increase our risk of dementia and cancer.

So, what has this LDL-C versus LDL-P discussion taught us? Very simply: *to measure your lipid health, measure your LDL particle count and don't focus solely on LDL-C.*[1]

Measuring Particles

In our highway analogy, the number of cars on our highway was the particle count. Analyzing your lipids to see the many classes of particles within the HDL and LDL categories is called *lipid subfraction analysis.* One of the major concepts in lipid subfraction analysis is that the *number* of LDL particles (LDL-P) is far more influential to cardiac health than the total amount of LDL (LDL-C). As the number of particles increases, the arteries become more and more crowded with particles. This increased particle density increases the opportunity for particles to diffuse into the walls of the coronary arteries. This is especially likely if the arterial walls

1. The very limited utility of LDL-C in measuring cardiac risk is compounded further when we learn that LDL-C isn't even measured in a standard cholesterol test. Instead, it's estimated using a very flawed calculation known as the Friedewald formula. See Appendix H for more information.

are brittle, cracked, thickened, and inflamed from high blood pressure, elevated glucose and insulin levels, and autoimmune attack.

Pioneering in the field of lipid subfraction analysis is LipoScience, a company that uses NMR (nuclear magnetic resonance) spectroscopy to examine the lipids and determine how many different types of particles are present. Companies such as LipoScience and their competitors are enabling researchers and physicians to better understand how lipid particles can be further classified, based upon size and density. I focus primarily on the LipoScience NMR in this discussion, largely because it is the one that I'm most familiar with. See *Testing Technologies* on page 45 for additional sources of lipid subfraction analysis.

As shown in the following illustration, LipoScience far more precisely measures lipid particle size and density than the traditional cholesterol test can.

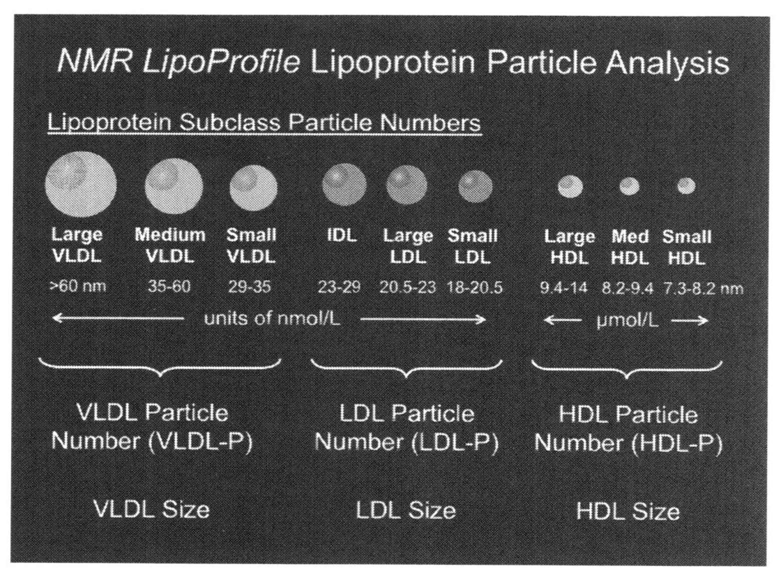

The NMR LipoProfile subfraction analysis. Image courtesy of LipoScience, Inc.

You don't really need to know what nmol/L or μmol/L means to know that a lower particle count is better. It's that simple when it comes to LDL particles.

Counting the Small Particles

In addition to identifying particle count, it's possible to identify which of the LDL particles are especially small in comparison to normal. This is important because many believe that egregiously small particles will more aggressively exploit cracks and fissures in the arterial walls, lodging there to become a breeding ground for cardiac plaque.

Lipidologists have been known to argue at conferences over which is more threatening to cardiac health: LDL total particle count or LDL small particle count. The former group says that the overall particle count is more of a risk because total particle count defines how much pressure is pushing the LDL particles into the arterial walls (much like a large number of people crammed into a subway car increases the chance of someone's face getting smashed against a wall, no matter how large or small the people are). The latter group says that small particle count is more of a factor because of the extremely small particles' tendency to more readily enter cracks and fissures in the arterial walls.

I say that both particle count *and* small particle count are a concern. A successful preventive health effort should address particle count *and* small particle count, just to be sure.

Particle Size

Related closely to *particle count* is *particle size*. As with the other factors, the various subfraction companies define particle size slightly differently but all agree: small particles = bad, large particles = good. This distinction is far more specific than just HDL v. LDL because even within the category of LDL, the larger LDL particles are considered by many researchers to not be harmful and likely even beneficial. Even with HDL, considered beneficial by all, larger HDL particles are more beneficial than small ones.

Other Players

Some other factors contribute to plaque formation: Lp-PLA2, homocysteine, and fibrinogen.

Lp-PLA2

Lp-PLA2 is an enzyme in the blood called *lipoprotein-associated phospholipase A2*. Lp-PLA2 causes arterial walls to be inflamed, increasing the risk of unstable, easily ruptured plaque.

One study showed that patients in the top 20% of Lp-PLA2 levels were twice as likely to have a heart attack as those in the bottom 20% of Lp-PLA2 levels, with all other factors being the same.[1]

Homocysteine

Homocysteine is a by-product of the metabolism of the essential amino acid methionine. There's some controversy surrounding homocysteine. It is known to correlate very well with cardiac risk because it promotes the formation of small, dense LDL particles,[2] and it helps the harmful Lp(a) molecules do their evil things (you will learn more about Lp(a) later). You can read more about homocysteine, and the difficulty in lowering it directly, in Chapter 7.

Fibrinogen

Fibrinogen is a sticky protein made by the liver and used in the body's clotting process. When levels of fibrinogen are elevated, it increases the risk of cardiac plaque formation and increases the risk of stroke and heart disease.[3]

Fibrinogen seems also to act in concert with Lp(a) to even further elevate the rate of plaque formation.[4]

A number of people report slightly lowering fibrinogen through exercise (and quitting smoking) but other than that, only certain antioxidants, primarily the spice *turmeric*, have been shown to effectively reduce fibrinogen.[5]

---

1. Packard, CJ, et al. Lipoprotein-associated phospholipase A2 as an independent predictor of coronary heart disease. West of Scotland Coronary Prevention Study Group. *New England Journal of Medicine* 2000 October 19;343(16):1148–1155.

2. Malinow, MR, et al. Carotid artery intimal-medial wall thickening and plasma homocyst(e)ine in asymptomatic adults. The Atherosclerosis Risk in Communities Study. *Circulation* 1993 April;87(4):1107–1113.

3. Danesh, J, et al. Plasma fibrinogen level and the risk of major cardiovascular diseases and nonvascular mortality: An individual participant meta-analysis. *JAMA* 2005 October 12;294(14):1799–1809.

4. Sechi, LA, De, MS. Relationship of lipoprotein(a) to variables of coagulation in hypertensive subjects. *Journal of Investigative Medicine* 2001 January;49(1):12–20.

5. Ramirez-Bosca, A., et al. An hydroalcoholic extract of Curcuma longa lowers the abnormally high values of human-plasma fibrinogen. *Mechanisms of Ageing and Development*, 2000,114:207–220.

The Cause of Unfavorable Lipid Particles

Even though I've spent time disputing the diet-health theory, diet does have an effect on our lipid profile and cardiovascular health. In fact, our diet is perhaps the single most influential factor in having favorable or unfavorable lipids, even more so than genetics. I believe this is true because human genetics have remained essentially unchanged for far more than the past half-century or so, yet the rates of cardiovascular disease have skyrocketed during this time, considerably more than can be attributed to improvements in cardiac diagnosis.

I believe those who benefit from selling statins love to say that genetics, not diet, has the most to do with cholesterol levels because doing so makes it easier to convince doctors, and subsequently their patients, that cholesterol level is beyond dietary control and everyone should therefore just take statins.

The "gotcha" here, though, is that if a person's lipid metabolism is broken from years of refined carbohydrates and vegetable oils, a statin may need to be part of the solution if diet and supplements don't bring the particle count down to a reasonable level.

Dietary Factors Affecting Lipids

The statin people have one thing right: When it comes to lipids, it's all about the liver. The liver, more than anything, controls the characteristics of the lipid particles in your body. We are therefore faced with the obvious question: What dietary factors affect the characteristics of the lipids that the liver produces?

This is a tough one.

If I knew the exact answers to this one, I'd probably win the Nobel Prize. We are all so diverse in so many ways that there may never be a single answer to the question of exactly how we should eat so that every single person produces ideal lipids.

Despite this uncertainty, some things very clearly affect the body unfavorably and should be avoided, the biggest culprit being wheat.

Wheat?

Yes, wheat.

According to Dr. Davis in his book *Wheat Belly*, wheat (even the exulted whole wheat) produces highly unfavorable lipid particles, sending particle counts up and particle size down. The ills associated with wheat are so numerous that I devote an entire section to wheat (and to my praises of *Wheat Belly*) below.

Another culprit in lipid health, and one that's sure to send your triglycerides skyward, is fructose, the "healthy" sugar that's in fruits and in "healthy" fruit juices.

Why is fructose so bad? The biggest reason is undoubtedly because fructose is metabolized directly by the liver (and not by an insulin response, like most sugars are), producing a host of unfavorable effects, including excess triglyceride production and, in the case of excessive fructose consumption, fatty liver disease.[1]

As you'll read in Chapter 3, controlling our glucose levels is vital to optimizing health and is a significant factor in the health of our liver. Elevated glucose levels in the bloodstream also disrupt the liver's performance, causing it to produce unfavorable lipid particles. Nothing increases blood glucose levels like carbohydrates, most significantly wheat, which typically increases blood glucose levels as high, or higher, than pure sucrose (table sugar).

Genetic Factors Affecting Lipids

Lp(a)

Some lipid particles, like HDL, are protective, and some, like small, dense LDL, are damaging. One particularly damaging lipid particle is known by the name *Lipoprotein(a)*, also called *Lp(a)*. Much has been written about Lp(a) and its role in heart disease, but for our purposes, we need to remember only that Lp(a) does nothing except stick where it shouldn't and that it very aggressively promotes cardiac plaque formation.

1. Ouyang, Xiaosen, et al. Fructose Consumption as a Risk Factor for Non-alcoholic Fatty Liver Disease. *Journal of Hepatolology* 2008 June;48(6): 993–999.

A person with high levels of Lp(a) has a greater risk of having vascular diseases, including vascular diseases of the brain (cerebrovascular disease), the peripheral limbs (peripheral vascular disease), and the heart (premature coronary artery disease).[1] One particularly frustrating thing about Lp(a) is that our levels seem to be greatly genetically influenced, which means that Lp(a) levels tend to remain at a relatively consistent level throughout our lifetime. There are, however, reports of people successfully lowering high Lp(a) levels with aggressive lifestyle changes and nutritional supplements as well as thyroid optimization.

If your Lp(a) levels are high, take this seriously, especially if you have a cardiac plaque issue. Do all the research you can on lowering your Lp(a) and be especially concerned about your lipid subfraction profiles because Lp(a) acts in concert with unfavorable lipid particles to aggressively form plaque. And don't believe those who tell you that there's nothing you can do to lower your Lp(a). It's true that lowering one's Lp(a) is tough to do, but many anecdotal reports show that it is possible.

Rather than spend countless pages on the many approaches people are taking to reduce Lp(a), I'll simply suggest that those of you with high Lp(a) levels spend some time on Dr. William Davis' online community, *TrackYourPlaque.com.* Track Your Plaque's membership is rich with cardiac health enthusiasts, many of whom have some very valuable insights into their own experiences in reducing Lp(a) levels through lifestyle changes.

ApoE

You may have read that drinking red wine will lower your risk of heart disease or that drinking red wine will increase your risk of heart disease. Equally valid studies show red wine to be helpful, neutral, or harmful to cardiovascular health.

This apparent discrepancy seems puzzling until you learn that the role of moderate alcohol intake on cardiovascular health appears to be genetically influenced. Based upon our genetics, a glass of red wine once a day may lower the risk of heart disease, may increase it, or may have no overall effect either way.

---

1. Berkeley HeartLab Clinical Reference Manual.

Similarly, our genetic tendencies can influence the way we metabolize certain saturated fats, with some genetic types more easily converting ingested saturated fats into favorable lipid particles and some not doing so quite as effectively.

How do we determine our individual genetics? How can we determine if we'll possibly benefit from a glass of red wine every day and if we're likely to produce favorable LDL particles when we ingest significant quantities of saturated fat? A simple *ApoE* genetic test can determine which genetic category you're in.

ApoE stands for *Apolipoprotein E.* Most people just refer to this gene as *ApoE.*

The three categories of ApoE are E2, E3, and E4. The implications of one's ApoE type and alcohol intake are as follows:[1]

E2 — Moderate alcohol intake tends to increase HDL and decrease LDL. E2 types are more likely to slightly decrease total LDL while increasing unfavorable LDL-P with a low-fat diet and be unaffected by a moderate fat diet. About 11% of the population falls into the E2 category.

E3 — Moderate alcohol intake tends to increase HDL. E3 types are more likely to moderately lower total LDL without affecting unfavorable LDL-P with a low-fat diet whereas a moderate fat diet tends to lower total LDL *and* lower unfavorable LDL-P. About 64% of the population falls into the E3 category.

E4 — Moderate alcohol intake tends to decrease HDL and increase LDL. E4 types are more likely to significantly lower total LDL and slightly lower unfavorable LDL-P with a low-fat diet and slightly lower total LDL while moderately increasing unfavorable LDL-P with a moderate fat diet. Approximately 25% of the population falls into the E4 category.

---

1. Berkeley HeartLab Clinical Reference Manual.

   Moderate alcohol intake is defined by the study authors to mean one drink per day for women and no more than two drinks per day for men. (Am J Clin Nutr 2001;73:736–45). Subsequent research has shown specific benefits from drinking red wine, which compels many of those who benefit from alcohol intake to confine themselves to drinking red wine.

Remember, though, that these are genetic *tendencies*, not *absolutes*. If, for example, you have caused yourself to become dyslipidemic from decades of excessive carbohydrate intake that has compromised your liver's ability to manufacture favorable lipid particles, you will likely respond very differently than your genetics suggests you might. A dyslipidemic E3, for example, who should be able to effectively metabolize saturated fats into favorable lipid particles, could behave more like an E4 and have an unfavorable response to excessive saturated fats. This is another reason why real-world experience and testing is more valuable to you in your search for an optimal lifestyle than any theoretical model, study, or opinion will predict. I can say this with confidence for I am one of E3 people who has a broken lipid metabolism and responds more like an E4, a fact that took monitoring my postprandial triglyceride levels to discover.

Note: The National Institute on Aging reports that researchers have also begun studying an apparent correlation between one's ApoE type and the risk of developing Alzheimer's disease, with the E4 type seeming to have the greatest risk. The reasons behind correlation are unclear, though many speculate that it has something to do with the formation of a certain type of plaque in the brain. Don't freak if you're ApoE E4, though. It doesn't mean that anything is guaranteed to happen. When researchers say "correlated" or "associated," it points to an interesting avenue for further research, not an absolute.

Testing Lipids in a Meaningful Way

What all of this information on lipids, subfraction analysis, and genetic markers means is that there's a much better way to examine your "cholesterol" than simply measuring the amount of cholesterol, or even HDL and LDL, in your blood. Taking cholesterol testing to the next level by measuring particle count, particle size, and various other factors like Lp(a) and LpPLA2 will dramatically increase the usefulness of your results.

Testing Technologies

A number of technologies are available for measuring lipid subfractions. Some physicians prefer one over another but ultimately any one of them is far more informative than a standard HDL/LDL test. Following are three sources of subfraction analysis that I'm familiar with:

LipoScience NMR — LipoScience is a great way to monitor lipid health. Ordering a LipoScience NMR to obtain my LDL particle number, LDL small particle number, and LDL size is easy and relatively affordable. I can order a LipoScience NMR online any time I want for about $100.

Atherotech VAP — The excellent VAP panel from Atherotech examines various subfractions of HDL and LDL and also includes the Lp(a) test, which is useful for identifying the presence of this highly damaging particle. The full VAP panel also includes vitamin D testing as well as a variety of inflammation markers and hormone levels.

Berkeley HeartLab — While not directly translatable to LipoScience's particle count and small particle count values or to the VAP's way of looking at things, the subfraction analysis from Berkeley HeartLab divides HDL into five size-based subcategories and LDL into seven size-based subcategories. Berkeley HeartLab's analysis is more expensive than the LipoScience NMR and the company's rules prohibit individuals from ordering the testing directly—only a physician can order an analysis from Berkeley HeartLab. Even though I find their analysis very useful and informative, the increased cost and inconvenience of going through my physician to obtain one means that I have a Berkeley HeartLab panel far less often than a LipoScience NMR.

Many people like running a LipoScience NMR and a VAP at the same time, believing that the two together provide an even better picture of lipid health. If cost weren't an issue, I'd run both a VAP and a LipoScience each time I check my lipids. However, what's most important is that you pick some method of monitoring your lipid subfractions and stick with it.

Goals for Your Lipid Subfraction Analysis

I'll talk more about specific numerical goals for lipid subfractions in Chapter 7, but basically we want our particle count to be low, our small particle count to be even lower, triglycerides to be low, and HDL to be high, all while maintaining a healthy amount of large, fluffy LDL.

To Recap: Why the HDL/LDL Model Is Overly Simplistic

The theory that eating cholesterol and fatty foods causes heart disease has paved the way for the opportunistic marketing of transfats, polyunsaturated fats (PUFAs), low-fat diets, and the carbohydrate-laden USDA food pyramid as well as to the demonization of healthy fats that served humankind well for millennia. Fortunately, this flawed theory has produced an ever-increasing number of highly respected critics, as discussed in more detail in Chapter 6.

The theory that high cholesterol levels in the blood cause heart disease is dangerously oversimplified in its stated context and has spawned a multi-billion dollar statin industry, fraught with misrepresentation and statistical sleight of hand.[1] The true story of how lipid levels in the blood affect our heart attack risk is far more complex and even though research is learning more every day, the data are very slow to reach the medical practitioners, the media, and the policy makers.

With what you now know about lipid subfraction analysis, you can see that trying to improve cardiac health by simply reducing LDL is like trying to reduce crime by jailing a random 75% of the people in the country. Sure, crime will go down because casting such a wide net will certainly capture a significant number of criminals, but the harm done by incarcerating a massive number of innocent individuals is incalculable.

The net result of all this lipid subfraction research is that we don't want to focus on the amount of cholesterol in our blood or even get tunnel vision on the HDL and LDL values alone. The bigger issues are how many lipid particles we have and what size they are, coupled with other factors in the body, like diabetes and inflammation.

---

1. See Appendix A for more information.

The Most Important Points from This Chapter

- Eating fat does not cause heart disease. In a great many cases, *avoiding fat* is what causes heart disease.
- Once you have heart disease, however, the picture becomes more complicated and highly variable, depending on the individual. For some battling heart disease, eating lots of fat is a good thing. For others, not so good. This is why trying to determine your optimal diet based upon studies or research articles that look at populations is very likely to fail.
- Trying to reduce your risk of heart disease by merely getting your LDL as low as possible can fail because it's not looking at the real problem, which is LDL particle count.
- The diet-health hypothesis that eating fat causes heart disease is wrong. The only kernels of truth are that excessive saturated fat intake, in the presence of elevated glucose levels, forms harmful Advanced Glycated End Products and that certain rare dyslipidemic people have trouble effectively metabolizing large amounts of saturated fats.
- The lipid hypothesis, which argues that high blood cholesterol levels cause heart disease, is wrong in its generality. When we look at lipid subfraction and examine particle count, small particle size, and other lipid subfactors, we learn that these factors (primarily LDL-P particle count), not total cholesterol, are the major culprits in lipid health.
- Statins have a role in combating heart disease but only in a very controlled way. Unilaterally prescribing statins to anyone with LDL-C over a certain number is simplistic, misguided, and dangerous.
- There are some genetic components to our lipid metabolism, but overall, carbohydrate intake (especially wheat) is the largest influence on the lipids that the liver produces.

If You Want to Take Action Immediately

- Speak with your physician about having a lipid subfraction analysis. If your physician is unwilling to order one for you, consider ordering a LipoScience NMR, a VAP, or both, from one of the companies online as described in the Appendix S.
- While you're ordering tests, also check your Lp-PLA2, homocysteine, and fibrinogen levels to determine a baseline for these key indicators.
- Have your Lp(a) checked to see if you need to concern yourself about this dangerous, plaque-promoting particle.
- Consider having your blood tested to see what ApoE genetic type you are, which may help you decide if a glass of red wine on a regular basis might be a good idea or a bad idea.

3

You're Probably Diabetic and Don't Even Know It

"Wait a minute!" I can almost hear you saying, "I don't need to take insulin. How can I possibly be a diabetic?"

It's no accident that diabetes is featured prominently in this book about preventive health. Diabetes is so pervasive in our country today that if you're over age forty, you have a significant chance of already being a diabetic.[1] Elevated glucose and insulin levels contribute significantly to most major diseases Americans face today. What's more alarming is that far more people are diabetic than realize it.

No matter your age or your history, do not skip this chapter just because you think there's no chance you could be diabetic. What you learn here may surprise you.

1. http://www.cdc.gov/diabetes/statistics/prev/national/tprevage.htm. According to the Centers for Disease Control and Prevention (CDC), 12% of Americans over the age of 45 have been diagnosed as diabetic. As you'll learn in this chapter, however, we are typically diabetic for many years before being diagnosed.

While most of us think of insulin syringes when we hear the term *diabetes*, diabetes simply means that our ability to make or utilize our natural insulin is compromised. Most people who could accurately be called diabetic have not progressed far enough in the disease process to require insulin—yet. That may sound like good news but it is not. You see, in the years, even decades, before diabetes becomes severe enough to require insulin, the diabetes has caused an extraordinary amount of damage to the body.

In fact, it could be argued that the greatest danger from diabetes is the harm that diabetes causes before it is detected.

This is not to minimize the serious, life-changing challenge that diabetes represents to those who have been diagnosed. Rather, it illustrates what an insidious and damaging disease diabetes is and how quietly it sneaks up on its unsuspecting victims.

Why must we be unsuspecting victims? If diabetes creeps up on us over years or even decades, why don't we have the technology to recognize diabetes well before it causes us harm? Why can't we detect diabetes in time to reverse the course of the disease so that we never suffer the harm that diabetes inflicts?

The sad truth is that we do have the technology to recognize the impending onset of Type 2 diabetes decades before it threatens us. Moreover, the technology to recognize that we are on a path to diabetes is cheap, easily accessible, and easy to use. Then why don't we?

Before we get into that, let's have an overview of glucose health and diabetes. This next section is a little long and technical, but bear with me. Understanding how the body metabolizes glucose and what can go wrong with that process is critical to the holistic concept of preventive medicine.

This chapter deals primarily with what's commonly called *Type 2* diabetes. For a discussion of the different types of diabetes, see Appendix C.

A Diabetes Primer

Most people know that glucose is the primary energy source for the body's cells and that glucose is transported into cells through the efforts of the hormone *insulin*, which is created by the beta cells of the pancreas. Without the presence of insulin, glucose cannot effectively enter the cells of the body and the cells will starve, no matter how much glucose is in the bloodstream. Insulin, therefore, is vital to maintaining the proper level of glucose in the cells and in the bloodstream.

Switching Fuel Sources to Maintain a Normal Glucose Level

Most of us take for granted that our next meal is readily available whenever we feel hungry or not long thereafter. For much of human history, however, eating regularly was by no means guaranteed.

Even though glucose is vital to the body's cells, it's ineffective for the body to try and store sizeable amounts of glucose as a fuel source—it's just too readily metabolized and not very energy-efficient. The body must have a long-term way of storing excess energy when glucose levels are high and quickly retrieving that stored energy when glucose levels are low. This is somewhat analogous to a hybrid car that can effortlessly switch from battery power to gasoline power and back again, as energy demands dictate.

The method the human body uses for storing excess energy is the fat cell, specialized cells that store fatty acids in our body. Fatty acids contain nearly twice as much energy per gram than glucose, making the fat cells effective storage sites for times when the body needs additional energy.

It's interesting to note that the number of fat cells is approximately equal in all body types—an obese person has about the same number of fat cells as a thin person. This is because fat cells can stretch to many times their original size, allowing them to contain significantly more fatty acids in one person than in another. You'll see later that the ability to move substances into and out of fat cells is an important part of our metabolism.

The body works very hard to ensure that glucose levels in the blood stay within a very narrow range, typically 70 to 80 mg/dL.[1] Too little glucose in the blood and the body experiences hypoglycemia, which is characterized by dizziness, unconsciousness, seizures, and possibly even brain damage and death. As any diabetic knows, the opposite problem, too much glucose in the bloodstream, is also very damaging, albeit in a slower, more progressive way, as it slowly causes kidney damage, nerve damage, blindness, heart disease, and loss of limbs.

Any time the glucose level in the body climbs higher than 80 mg/dL or so, the body must metabolize that glucose quickly. This means releasing the hormone *insulin*, which, when released into the bloodstream will do the following:

- Cause the fat in the bloodstream to be pulled into fat cells so that the glucose, and not the fat, will be metabolized.
- Activate the glucose receptors on the cell membranes so that the cells can begin pulling glucose into the cells for energy.

When the cells have metabolized the glucose and the glucose level in the bloodstream drops into the normal range, the insulin level drops as well. The lowered insulin levels then tell the body to release fat from the fat cells so that the body can use fat as an energy source, a process called gluconeogenesis, the conversion of non-carbohydrates into glucose. In a healthy, non-diabetic person, the body switches effortlessly back and forth between using glucose for energy and using fat for energy, shuffling fat into and out of the fat cells, as needed, to maintain blood glucose levels in a healthy, narrow range.

Understanding this glucose and insulin-controlled switch between energy sources is fundamental to understanding why we feel hungry at certain times and what foods promote health versus what foods degrade health.

A Bag of Chips and a 64-Ounce Soda

Let's think about the amount of glucose in a healthy, non-diabetic person. In such a person, the total amount of glucose in the blood-

---

1. mg/dL means "milligrams per deciliter," and in the United States is the most common measurement of glucose concentration in the blood.

stream during the fasting state is less than a teaspoon (which is less than 4 grams of glucose). An 80-pound, fasting, non-diabetic child has less than one-half teaspoon of glucose.

A 64-ounce soda can contain over 200 grams of sucrose. Sucrose is 50% glucose and 50% fructose.

A 64-ounce cup of soda can contain over 200 grams of sucrose. Sucrose is 50% glucose and 50% fructose. What do you think happens when a person eats a meal that dumps ten or a hundred times the fasting amount of sugar into the bloodstream? The body simply cannot allow the blood glucose level to suddenly become 100 times the normal fasting amount. That much glucose in the bloodstream would be acutely harmful, perhaps even fatal, if not metabolized quickly. The body reacts to elevated glucose levels by doing whatever it must do to quickly metabolize the glucose. This means secreting insulin. Lots of insulin! Way more insulin than was ever necessary for a person before the advent of refined white flour, 64-ounce sodas, tortilla chips, and candy bars.

What? Speak Up! I Can't Hear You!

When sugar-laden meals repeatedly cause a bunch of insulin to flood the body, the large amounts of glucose seeking entrance into the cells become overwhelming to the glucose receptors on the cell membranes. From their perspective, it's as though someone suddenly started screaming at them, so they cover their ears. (In biochemistry parlance, the glucose receptors *down-regulate.*) It's no different from when you fry a pan of odorous fish in your kitchen and stink up the whole house. After a while, you barely notice the smell. This isn't because the odor has dissipated. The odor is less noticeable because you have become desensitized to the smell. If you left the house and spent a short time in fresh air, you would undoubtedly smell the fish again far more intensely when you returned.

Over time and with frequent exposure to high levels of insulin, the cells in the body become increasingly resistant to insulin, requiring more and more insulin to accomplish the same glucose transport functions as before. Just like a person becoming increasingly deaf, the cells require that insulin speak louder and louder as their insulin resistance increases. Finally, as the cells' ability to respond to insulin become increasingly weakened, the cells can literally starve, even though more than ample glucose is present in the bloodstream around them.

The Effects of Insulin Resistance

Today's typical diet is causing virtually all of us to become increasingly insulin-resistant as we age. One visible side effect of insulin resistance is weight gain. While weight gain is frequently what our society focuses on, the harmful effects of insulin resistance are considerably more than just losing our trim figures. Moreover, for those people who are actively trying to lose weight, the weight gain itself isn't the most difficult obstacle to overcome—it's the inability to pull fat out of the fat cells in time of need. When a non-insulin-resistant person skips a meal or eats an unusually small portion, the body easily makes up the difference by pulling fat out of fat cells for more energy. In contrast, when an insulin-resistant person skips a meal, the higher insulin levels in the body keep the fat trapped in the fat cells and the other cells literally starve, even though the body has a fuel source nearby.

It may seem unbelievable that having an elevated fasting insulin level could prevent the body from burning fat when we're hungry, but it's true. Insulin is amazingly powerful at keeping fat locked into fat cells where it remains inaccessible and cannot be metabolized for energy. How powerful? Obese rats that are given insulin injections to maintain high insulin levels and then put on a starvation diet remained obese while dying of starvation. These starving, yet obese rats *digested their own muscles and organs for food* until they died from starvation, *without losing any of their body fat.*

Yes, even though they were starving, the elevated insulin levels prevented their body from metabolizing fat from their fat cells for energy, forcing their bodies to digest their own organs and muscles for nourishment. Think about this the next time you wonder why people can't lose their unwanted body fat even though they are not eating much. It's very likely that the foods that they are eating are causing a large insulin response, which is keeping the fat locked into their fat cells.

As the cells in an overweight, insulin-resistant person cry out for energy, the dieter feels the crushing pain of hunger and has little choice but to eat. Unfortunately, they frequently choose a "healthy, low-fat" snack like a turkey sandwich on whole grain bread, rice cakes, baked potato, pasta, or perhaps a piece of fruit or a bowl of popcorn. What happens then? Such dieters feel full immediately after eating, but because they ate foods that are high in carbohydrates, their postprandial glucose levels have once again spiked well beyond the healthy 70 to 80 mg/dL range, perhaps as high as 150 mg/dL or more, causing the body to produce—what?—a bunch of insulin. The insulin works as hard as it can to reduce the glucose level to a non-harmful range, and in doing so, further traps the fat in the body's fat cells. The glucose receptors in the body become even more desensitized as the body experiences more and more episodes of large, glucose-producing meals, causing them increasingly greater difficulty in metabolizing the glucose that frequently floods the bloodstream.[1]

The net result of this vicious cycle is that the insulin-resistant dieter is starving again in a few hours when cells are once again hungry for the glucose that they cannot metabolize well. And worse, such individuals are prohibited by the high insulin levels from metabolizing the fat they so desperately want to shed.

And instead of occasionally experiencing blood glucose and insulin levels that are harmfully high, the insulin-resistant person spends the majority of his or her time with glucose levels in the triple-digit range and with insulin levels that are elevated to harmful levels. This is especially true if they are following the typical "healthy" advice to eat lots of grains, avoid fat, and eat small frequent meals.

Fat or Thin, Dieting or Not—Insulin Resistance Doesn't Care

The most surprising thing about the effect of insulin resistance and trapping fat in fat cells is that despite what I've just said about this effect, we cannot determine how insulin-resistant we are by how much extra fat we are carrying. While it's true that an overweight person is almost certainly insulin-resistant, a thin person is no less likely so. Why is this? It's because fat cells can become insulin resistant at different times in different people. If you're "lucky"

---

1. Another impediment to proper glucose receptor function is overindulging in omega-6 fatty acids. Left with no choice, the body uses omega-6 fatty acids to repair cell membranes, damaging and impeding the receptors that are embedded within. Read more about omega-6 fatty acids in Chapter 4.

enough to have fat cells that become insulin resistant quickly, before they expand considerably, then you're a thin, insulin-resistant person, subject to the same damage from elevated glucose and insulin levels as an obese insulin-resistant person. Everything I've said in this section about fat being trapped in fat cells and about a person becoming hungry every couple of hours and spending the majority of the time with elevated glucose and insulin levels can be just as true for a thin person as for an overweight person. In fact, it's probably the thin person who is less fortunate when it comes to insulin resistance because the thin, insulin-resistant person's diabetes will go undetected far longer, due to the false sense of security that being thin brings.

The Myth of Eating Frequent Meals

Many well-meaning nutritionists tell diabetics (or those at risk of being diabetic) to eat small, frequent meals instead of large meals. This, in my opinion, is frequently horribly misguided advice, especially when coupled with the typical recommendation to get 60–65% of one's calories from grains, which considerably elevate blood glucose levels.

Think about this: If the food these insulin-resistant people are eating is causing their blood glucose and insulin levels to rise to unfavorable levels every time they eat, what would be the effect of eating small, frequent meals? The answer is simple: They would remain in a state of elevated glucose and insulin levels for essentially all of their waking hours. By the time their body finishes metabolizing the glucose from a high carbohydrate meal, they eat another meal, sending their glucose level right back into an unfavorable range. The recommendation to eat small, frequent meals is nothing more than an attempt to help people deal with feelings of hunger every two hours, the result of the typical modern meal that causes the insulin-resistant among us to feel hungry two hours after eating an unhealthy, carbohydrate-laden meal. The net effect of this misguided dietary advice is to very effectively train us to graze all day like farm animals, keeping our blood glucose and insulin levels elevated for all our waking hours.

And we wonder why we're a nation of overweight Type 2 diabetics?

It's actually pretty simple: If you're hungry every two hours, something is wrong with the way you're eating.

A better approach for controlling our blood glucose is to eat fewer meals and try to compress them into the shortest timeframe possible. Instead of eating 16 hours a day and fasting 8 hours a day, it's much better for our glucose metabolism to eat 8 hours a day and fast 16. More fasting time means more time with lowered blood glucose and insulin levels and more time that allows our insulin-resistant bodies to heal.

It's No Longer Called *Adult Onset Diabetes*

The term *adult onset diabetes*, as Type 2 diabetes was once called, has fallen into disuse because of dramatically increasing rates of Type 2 diabetes among children and teens. Indeed, once rare among the young, Type 2 diabetes is now common.[1] Insulin resistance can even begin developing even before birth if the mother's diet promotes excessive insulin production. And by the teens and early 20s, the effects of insulin resistance are already quite apparent and have begun damaging the body.

Insulin resistance begins happening decades before symptoms appear and is an underlying factor in nearly every malady that we struggle with as adults.

What Other Harm Comes from Insulin Resistance?

From all the talk about insulin and glucose, you probably think that metabolizing glucose is insulin's only role. It's not. In fact, many physicians and researchers believe that metabolizing glucose is a very minor role for insulin. They believe that because of our modern diets, composed of far more sugars and starches than in past centuries, glucose has become known primarily for glucose metabolism when, in fact, insulin does far more than just regulating glucose. Insulin's primary role in the body is actually as a growth hormone.

1. Pinhas-Hamiel O, et al. Increased incidence of non-insulin dependent diabetes mellitus among adolescents. *Journal of Pediatrics* 1996;128:608–615.

Insulin is one of the oldest known growth hormones, first identified in the early 1900s. Throughout the cells of the body are growth hormone receptors that respond to growth hormones by instructing the cell to grow. Growth hormones in the body are referred to as IgFs, or *insulin-like growth factors*, because of their similarity to the grandfather of all growth hormones, insulin. In fact, insulin is such an effective growth hormone that some body builders purchase and inject insulin to help grow muscle tissue more quickly. (For the record, this sounds like a really bad idea to me.)

Perhaps the biggest problem with insulin being a growth hormone is that not all of the tissues in the body become desensitized to increasing levels of insulin at the same rate. As a person becomes more and more insulin-resistant, cells that are much less affected continue to respond to the ever-increasing levels of insulin, growing and multiplying more rapidly as insulin levels increase. What cells exhibit this behavior? The endothelial cells that form the lining of your arteries, for one. As these arterial cells multiply more rapidly, the lining of an insulin-resistant person's arteries thicken and grow inward, hastening coronary artery disease. This is one of the reasons why so many diabetics die from heart disease.

Insulin levels also have considerable effect on the thyroid. The thyroid produces T4, which is a hormone that needs to be converted to T3 before it can be effectively used by the body. This conversion of T4 to T3 primarily occurs in the liver. When the liver becomes insulin-resistant, the liver no longer effectively converts T4 to T3, which causes hypothyroidism. Hypothyroidism, in turn, disrupts the effectiveness of the liver, causing the liver to produce unfavorable lipid particles, discussed more fully in Chapter 2.

When insulin levels increase, the blood in the body clots more readily, increasing the risk of heart attack and stroke. In addition, macrophage (a type of white blood cell) levels increase, hastening the formation of cardiac plaque.[1] In fact, researchers believe that macrophages are the predominant cells involved in the formation of plaque lesions in coronary arteries.[2]

---

1. Liang C-P, et al. The macrophage at the crossroads of insulin resistance and atherosclerosis. *Circulation Research* 2007;100;1546–1555.

2. Lucas AD, Greaves DR. Atherosclerosis: Role of chemokines and macrophages. *Expert Reviews in Molecular Medicine* 2001;3(25):1–18.

As if coronary artery disease wasn't bad enough, research shows very clearly that insulin levels show some of the strongest correlations with colon and breast cancer. This is because cancer cells have a profound affinity for glucose. In fact, cancer cells have so much affinity for glucose that certain cancer detection scans employ a special radioactive form of glucose that the scanner can detect. Bright spots on the image are places where cells have gobbled up very high levels of the radioactive glucose. These areas of high glucose consumption are the cells that are flagged as more likely to be cancerous.

High insulin levels also increase the excretion of magnesium and calcium in the urine, causing a deficiency in magnesium and a loss of calcium. Furthermore, high insulin levels cause the calcium that remains in the body to be deposited incorrectly, not in the bones where it belongs, but in the coronary arteries. Increasing calcium intake isn't always a good idea because studies show that women who supplement with calcium are twice as likely to have a heart attack.[1] Because insulin also damages nerve cells, many diabetics suffer from neuropathy, a chronic and debilitating condition. The most commonly damaged nerve is the vagus nerve, the largest nerve in the body. Running from the head to the lower extremities, the vagus nerve is a principal component in a person's *parasympathetic nervous system*, which controls the involuntary functions of your body, that is, the things that happen without your thinking about them.

Your heart rate and digestive functions are two examples of things that your parasympathetic nervous system handles without your conscious thought. A damaged vagus nerve brings a variety of complications, including irregular and abnormal heart rates and delayed digestion (known as *gastroparesis*). Gastroparesis causes dramatically delayed stomach emptying and poor digestion, which results in acid reflux, constipation, diarrhea, and cramping. Very slow digestion can also cause unhealthy bacteria to flourish in the digestive system, further impeding nutrient absorption, worsening acid reflux, and even interfering with thyroid function. Because 20% of the thyroid hormone T4 is converted to the more useful

1. Bolland MJ, et al. Vascular events in healthy older women receiving calcium supplementation: Randomised controlled trial. *British Medical Journal*, 2008;336(7638):262–266.

hormone T3 by the healthy bacteria in the gut, disrupting gut health can cause hypothyroidism, which disrupts the liver, causing the liver to produce the wrong kind of lipids, which causes heart disease.

Nerves damaged by high glucose levels cause a variety of symptoms in the extremities, too, as limbs slowly lose the ability to respond properly to their surroundings or to effectively report feelings of pain and temperature. The results of this include numbness and pain in the hands and feet, as well as loss of muscle strength and control. The increased occurrence of ulcers and infections among diabetics, especially in the extremities, frequently results in amputation.

Perhaps one of the most unfortunate effects of insulin resistance is the damage that it does to the pancreas, thus worsening insulin resistance. This happens because high levels of glucose in the blood kill pancreatic beta cells, the cells responsible for producing insulin. As more beta cells die, the ability of the pancreas to produce insulin is even further compromised, thus increasing glucose levels even more. Then, because there are fewer beta cells to handle the workload, the remaining beta cells must work harder and thereby die more quickly, thus completing this vicious cycle of beta cell destruction. And like a freight train gaining momentum, it's much more difficult to slow this progress of destruction the longer it's been accelerating.

Remember, there's no magic switch thrown when a doctor suddenly pronounces that a person is diabetic. The damage I've described happens over a long period of time, long before the condition has deteriorated enough to be officially called a diabetic. Therefore, the person at risk for these diabetic complications could very easily be you if your glucose level routinely gets high enough to be damaging, a point that will be clear very soon.

How High Is Too High?

Optimal fasting glucose levels are typically between 70 and 80 mg/dL. Just how high do glucose levels need to be before beta cells begin to die?

Much lower than you think.

One group of researchers has identified exposure to 140 mg/dL or higher as being deadly to beta cells.[1] Others have discovered that beta cell death begins whenever blood glucose levels exceed 100 mg/dL.[2]

Some studies say damage begins at glucose levels of 120 mg/dL, some at 110 mg/dL, and some even say anything over 90 mg/dL is harmful. The precise line where damage begins will likely differ slightly, depending upon the individual, but no matter which of these levels we choose, it's certain that today's typical diet of sugar, whole grains, pastas, potatoes, sodas, and snacks is routinely sending our blood glucose levels way beyond any reasonable limit.

If You Only Remember One Thing from This Chapter, Remember This

Every single moment that your blood glucose is elevated, your body is suffering harm!

THINK YOU'RE EATING HEALTHY? TAKE THIS CHALLENGE

However you're choosing to eat, be it a structured diet like the Zone Diet, Weight Watchers, Slim for Life, or if you're just "eating healthy most of the time," there's a fantastic way to determine if your diet is causing harm: Go to the drugstore and buy a glucose meter and a box of 50 test strips.

Read the instructions and learn how to properly use your meter (it's very simple and will only take a few minutes to learn). Then, for the next week, test your blood glucose level before eating and one hour and two hours after finishing each meal.

If your one-hour and two-hour blood glucose levels never exceed 110 mg/dL or so, congratulations, you're likely eating in such a way as to avoid causing damaging blood glucose spikes.

---

1. Gleason, CE, et al. Determinants of glucose toxicity and its reversibility in pancreatic islet Beta-cell line, HIT-T15. *American Journal of Physiology, Endocrinology, and Metabolism* 2000;279: E997–E1002.

2. Gastaldelli, A, et al. Beta-cell dysfunction and glucose intolerance: results from the San Antonio metabolism (SAM) study. *Diabetologia* 2004 Jan;47(1):31–39.

If, on the other hand, you're routinely seeing blood glucose levels of 130 mg/dL or 150 or even 200, then your diet is causing harmful levels of glucose in your body and is speeding you toward Type 2 diabetes.

Why Is Diabetes Undiagnosed for So Long?

If high insulin levels are harmful to so many systems in the body, then why is it so easy for this harm to go unnoticed and for diabetes to remain undiagnosed for so long?

The answer to that question is complicated and is a product of a number of factors, including human nature and economics.

As Jenny Ruhl writes in her very compelling book, *Blood Sugar 101*, back before diabetes was as controllable as it is today, a diagnosis of diabetes was quite nearly a death sentence. It was common for those diagnosed with diabetes to instantly be fired from their jobs, be denied life insurance, and find their health insurance canceled. The medical entities setting the guidelines for defining diabetes recognized this and made the requirements for being classified as a diabetic rather strict, so as to prevent borderline or pre-diabetics from being classified as diabetic and facing the stigma of the disease. Unfortunately, even though attitudes toward the disease have radically changed since then, these guidelines are much the same now as they were then, frequently delaying the diagnosis of diabetes. As a result, physicians and patients are typically very slow to admit that intervention and lifestyle changes are necessary, often until an unfortunate level of damage has occurred.

Another factor delaying an effective diagnosis of diabetes is likely denial. Nobody wants to be labeled a diabetic, especially someone whose only symptom is mildly elevated fasting glucose. Most people simply don't want to solve a problem while it's still far off in the distance. They'd rather wait until the problem is unequivocal and acute before taking action. This is most unfortunate because the earlier a person starts making lifestyle changes, the easier it is to prevent or reverse Type 2 diabetes.

Further thwarting effective diabetes diagnosis is the nature of the tests being used today. The gold standard test used to be the oral glucose tolerance test, a test in which doctors measure a patient's blood glucose levels over a period of hours following the ingestion of a measured amount of glucose. This test very effectively shows how well a patient is able to metabolize glucose, which is at the very core of defining diabetes. The moderate expense of the oral glucose tolerance test, unfortunately, is causing it to be displaced in favor of a cheaper fasting glucose test, where a single glucose measurement of a patient's fasting glucose level is used to define whether a patient is diabetic. Unfortunately, as you'll read later, of all the measurements of glucose metabolic health, an elevated fasting glucose is typically the last laboratory indicator to show diabetes. By basing a diagnosis of diabetes solely on fasting glucose, the diagnosis is typically delayed until a life-altering amount of damage has occurred. Similarly, as shown later in this chapter, the A1C test, which is just an estimate of a patient's average glucose levels for the preceding 100 days, is fraught with a variety of limitations, making it also a much less effective tool for defining whether one is diabetic.

How Do We Measure the Health of Our Glucose Metabolism?

By now it's clear that being insulin-resistant means being a Type 2 diabetic. It should also be clear that insulin resistance in Type 2 diabetics develops over time, sometimes decades.

> It's so cheap and easy to effectively measure your risk of diabetes on a regular basis that it's simply foolish not to do so.

This slow progression of the disease affords us the opportunity to recognize that we're on the path to diabetes well before our outcome is inevitable. While there are a number of tests that will show when we are clearly a diabetic, recognizing the signs of impending diabetes years or decades away typically requires a combination of tests and a deeper understanding of their implications than most people have.

Earlier in the chapter I talked about how easy it is to test yourself for diabetes and even to test to see if the way you're eating is putting you at risk for developing diabetes decades in the future. Unfortunately, your self-testing isn't likely to impress your doctor unless the standard tests that he or she is accustomed to performing also show a problem. The diabetes tests most commonly run by physicians during standard testing are A1C, fasting insulin, fasting glucose, and oral glucose tolerance test. First, I'll describe each of these and explain their implications and then show how they all tie together to form a big picture of how firmly you've placed yourself on the path to Type 2 diabetes.

Finally, I'll talk about what conventional medical wisdom says about the results and how waiting until your doctor or the American Diabetes Association says that you are diabetic means waiting until the disease is irreversible and perhaps life-threatening.

The A1C Test

Most people know what oxidation is—a substance reacting with oxygen. But most people aren't familiar with the term glycation. Glycation is nothing more than the process of a substance bonding with sugar (glucose).

Whenever a red blood cell in your bloodstream encounters a glucose molecule, there is a certain probability that the two will combine. The more glucose that is present in your bloodstream, the more opportunity there is for a glucose molecule and a red blood cell to bond, forming a glycated hemoglobin molecule. By measuring the percentage of red blood cells in a blood sample that have become glycated, it is a straightforward procedure to estimate what your average blood glucose level has been over the lifespan of an average red blood cell, which is typically 90 to 100 days. This is a useful indicator of whether your dietary habits have set you on a path toward Type 2 diabetes.

The A1C test is very inexpensive and very accessible. There are three common ways to get an A1C test.

- Ask your doctor to order it for you. This method has the advantage of involving your physician in the test, possibly affording the opportunity to discuss the results with a healthcare professional and form a strategy.
- Purchase the test online yourself and have it done at LabCorp. Many people don't know that they can order virtually any blood test online, pay a very reasonable price for it, and have the blood drawn at the same LabCorp facility that their doctor

would send them to. The A1C test, purchased online and performed at LabCorp, will cost somewhere around $50. See Appendix S for more information.

- Buy a home A1C testing kit that requires you to place a spot of blood on a specific type of card and send it to a lab. While some reports indicate that many home testing kits are unacceptably inaccurate,[1] Heritage Labs International, contracted by Walmart at the time of this writing, is reported by one independent study to have accuracy equal to that of the standard, LabCorp-type serum A1C tests. For less than $10, you can purchase a home A1C testing kit and receive your results within a few days.

What Does Your A1C Result Mean?

Recall that the A1C result is reported as a percentage of the red blood cells that have bonded to a glucose molecule.

Using a common formula, you can convert this A1C percentage to a value that represents an *estimate* of your average glucose value over the past 90 to 100 days. One of the most commonly used formulas is:

Mean plasma glucose = (35.6 x A1C) - 77.3.

Let's say that you had an A1C blood test result of 5.6%. Using this formula, an A1C value of 5.6 would calculate to an estimated *average* glucose value of 122 mg/dL.

From the diabetes primer section, you know that glucose levels higher than 110 or 120 are harmful, even if they last only a few hours at a time.

What will your A1C result be? 4.5? 5.0? 6.0? Higher?

If you are someone with an A1C result that translates to an average glucose level of greater than 100 or so, then you know for certain that no matter what you think about the merits of your diet, you have not been eating in such a way as to prolong your health. The higher the A1C value, the more damage you've been

---

1. Lenters-Westra, E, Slingerland, RJ. Six of eight hemoglobin A1C point-of-care instruments do not meet the general accepted analytical performance criteria. *Clinical Chemistry* 2010;56:1, 44–52.

doing and the faster you are propelling yourself toward Type 2 diabetes.

Don't be reassured if your A1C says that your average glucose level is below 100 or 110, either. Remember, the A1C value gives you an estimate of your *average* blood glucose, not your *maximum*. Because glucose levels fluctuate as much as 50 or 100 mg/dL (or more for people on high glycemic diets), for you to have an average glucose level of 110, you would need to spend a significant amount of time with a glucose level *above* 110.

Using just an A1C test, you can only speculate how much higher than average you went and how long you stayed there. If you know your fasting glucose level, the picture becomes somewhat clearer because the fasting glucose defines the lowest glucose levels you experience and the A1C provides a reasonable estimate of the average. We'll talk more about the fasting glucose level and its implication shortly.

Limitations to the A1C Test

The A1C test is useful, but it is far from perfect. It has a number of shortcomings that you should keep in mind when you are evaluating the results.

- Statistically, the A1C test gives a somewhat accurate average glucose level, but it's only an estimate. Your true average glucose level could be significantly higher or lower than the average value calculated from the A1C. Why the difference? Because the conversion is done using a mathematical formula that was derived by having a quantity of people test their glucose levels regularly, then testing their A1C value. Using the A1C values from this sample group, researchers created a mathematical formula for estimating any person's average glucose level based upon the individual's A1C value. As with most any test performed on a group of people, individual results will vary, sometimes significantly. As a result, the most commonly used formula for converting A1C to average glucose levels has an error of plus or minus 20%, meaning that an average blood glucose reported to be 154 mg/dL could actually be anywhere from 123 to 185 mg/dL.[1] This is quite a difference for a test that's being used to determine whether a person is diabetic.

There are other A1C conversion formulas, each producing slightly different calculated average blood glucose values. All such formulas, however, are subject to the same statistical errors because they are all created from a mathematical model that is derived from a sample of patient data. The implications of this margin for error and its implications for recommendations from the American Diabetes Association are discussed on page 76.

- A given glucose level must last for a while before it is reflected in the A1C. For example, if you eat a high sugar meal and your glucose level exceeds 200 mg/dL for only a few hours afterwards, the effect of that meal is not likely to be reflected in the A1C value, even though a glucose level that high will still be causing significant harm to your body.
- The National Glycohemoglobin Standardization Program cautions that consuming significant quantities of vitamin C will result in an inaccurate A1C value.
- Because the A1C value is affected by the lifespan of the red blood cells, any condition or activity that shortens the effective lifespan of your red blood cells will affect the A1C. For example, donating blood or being slightly anemic.
- Because high glucose levels hasten red blood cell death, reducing (improving) your blood glucose levels will *increase* the lifespan of red blood cells. This means that as you change your diet and lifestyle to produce lower blood glucose levels, your red blood cells live *longer*, which gives them *more* time to bond with a glucose molecule, thus *increasing* your A1C value.

  Huh?

  Yes, it seems counterintuitive but it makes sense. Think about it this way: Cheech the beachcomber walks the beach every day. Even though Cheech's reckless lifestyle of drinking and wrestling sharks will pretty much ensure he won't live past 35, because ol' Cheech spends nearly every day walking along the

---

1. Range reported is for a 95% confidence interval. Nathan, DM, et al. Translating the A1C assay into estimated average glucose values. *Diabetes Care* 2008:31:1473–1478.

> water, there's a given chance that he'll be pooped on by a seagull at some point during his rather short lifetime.
>
> What do you think will happen if Cheech suddenly gives up drinking, stops wrestling sharks, and starts taking vitamins every day? His lifespan will increase. He will have more time to spend on the beach, which means a greater likelihood of being pooped on by a seagull during his lifetime. The same is true for a red blood cell: A longer life span means the red blood cell has more chance of being pooped on by a glucose molecule before it dies.
>
> While typically not enough to offset the lowered A1C from improved glucose levels, this increased red blood cell lifespan *can* reduce the accuracy of the A1C value somewhat.

As you can see, the A1C is affected upwards or downward by a variety of factors, producing a value that's useful but far from perfect. This, coupled with the inherent margin of error in the conversion formula itself, causes me to grow increasingly concerned at pressures from insurance companies and other entities to use A1C as a sole indicator of diabetes risk.

Fasting Insulin

You'll recall from the diabetes primer that the body will always try to maintain glucose levels in an ideal range. As the body becomes more and more resistant to the insulin, however, the body will require increasing amounts of insulin to maintain this optimal blood glucose level. The fasting insulin level is an important indicator of glucose health because it shows us just how hard our body needs to work to maintain a given fasting glucose level.

Think about these two hypothetical individuals:

- A person with fasting glucose of 85 mg/dL and fasting insulin level of 15 uUI/mL[1]
- A person with the same fasting glucose level of 85 mg/dL and a fasting insulin level of only 4 uUI/mL.

1. uUI/mL stands for "microunits of insulin per milliliter" and is the standard measurement of insulin level in the bloodstream.

All other things being equal, the first person is further along the path toward Type 2 diabetes because he or she needs nearly four times the insulin as the second person to metabolize glucose with the same effectiveness. The most important message from this example is that even if two people have the same fasting glucose, their fasting insulin levels can differ, depending on how insulin-resistant their bodies are.

Fasting Glucose

Even if we haven't eaten in a while, the body will still produce glucose to feed itself. This basal level of glucose is present to fuel the cells as they perform routine functions. You may remember from earlier in this chapter that a healthy, non-diabetic person effortlessly switches from metabolizing glucose in the bloodstream to metabolizing fats from the fat cells as the body's demands and fasting state dictate. The ultimate goal of this glucose metabolism "machine" is to maintain glucose levels in a narrow, healthy range. If the glucose level is too high, the body attempts to lower it. If the glucose level is too low, the body attempts to raise it.

The net effect of insulin resistance is that glucose levels in the body creep upwards over time, despite the increased presence of insulin trying to maintain glucose levels in a narrow range.

A healthy, non-diabetic person's fasting glucose should be in or near the range of 70 to 80 mg/dL. Years of eating foods that induce insulin resistance will typically cause fasting glucose levels in the 90 to 100 mg/dL range around the age 40, with fasting glucose levels growing even higher as we continue to age. As you know, glucose levels above 110 mg/dL or so, even for a short time, will likely damage the body's systems. Having a fasting glucose level of 90 or 100 mg/dL means that the body doesn't have much "ceiling" or cushion to allow for increases in glucose levels after eating. That "healthy" breakfast consisting of a slice of wheat toast, low-fat yogurt, a banana, and a glass of orange juice is likely sending such a person's glucose close to 150 or even 200 mg/dL within an hour or two, causing damaging glucose spikes and elevated insulin levels, every single day.

The biggest problem with the fasting glucose test is not the test itself, but rather the fact that some use the fasting glucose test alone to assess the risk of diabetes. You'll learn more later about why relying on the fasting glucose test is ill-advised.

Oral Glucose Tolerance Test

The oral glucose tolerance test used to be the gold standard of diabetes diagnosis tools. Very simply, an oral glucose tolerance test requires ingesting a specific amount of glucose (usually 75 grams, all at once); then the blood is drawn at regular intervals (typically hourly) for a period of two, four, or six hours. The level of the person's blood glucose at specific time intervals after eating a known quantity of glucose is a very useful indicator of a person's glucose metabolism, with the two-hour glucose level being the most valuable.

For a number of reasons, the oral glucose tolerance test is becoming less commonly used, in favor of the A1C test. Here's why:

- The A1C test is much cheaper and more convenient, requiring only a single blood draw and analysis and not requiring fasting
- The oral glucose tolerance test is a huge assault on the body, especially on a patient with advanced Type 2 diabetes or heart disease, sometimes sending the glucose level above 200 mg/dL.

A very useful, but rarely used, alternative to the oral glucose tolerance test is called the *insulin challenge*, wherein a physician administers a given quantity of insulin intravenously and measures how much the patient's blood glucose drops over time. While this is much less stress on the body than the glucose tolerance test, the risk of hypoglycemia (low blood sugar) and the need for very close, careful monitoring compels most physicians to avoid the insulin challenge.

The Big Picture: What Do All These Diabetes Tests Mean?

The Progression of Type 2 Diabetes

To put these diabetic assessment tests in perspective, let's look at the typical way that Type 2 diabetes progresses.[1]

1. First, diet and lifestyle choices cause routinely elevated glucose levels in the body. This begins happening as early as childhood for those frequently fed foods like refined flour, grains (even whole grains), sugar, and starches (potatoes, pasta).

   These elevated postprandial glucose levels would be revealed by an inexpensive home glucose meter decades before one becomes an insulin-dependent diabetic.

2. Over time, the routinely elevated glucose levels cause the cells to become insulin-resistant and, as a result, the pancreas needs to create much more insulin to maintain the same glucose levels, fasting and non-fasting. This increased demand is placing a heavy burden on the pancreatic beta cells, the cells of the pancreas that are responsible for producing insulin. Burdened in this manner, beta cells die much more quickly than if they were responding to more moderate glucose demands. Fasting insulin begins to rise at this point.

   Fasting insulin, largely ignored in a routine physical, would provide years more warning than fasting glucose levels that Type 2 diabetes is looming.

3. After years or decades of Steps 1 and 2, the patient's cells are so resistant to insulin and so many pancreatic beta cells have died that the pancreas can no longer keep up with the demands placed upon it. At this point as much as 50% of the beta cells in the patient's pancreas are dead, perhaps even

1. This progression deals only with the effects of a high glycemic diet on development of Type 2 diabetes. While a high glycemic diet is the largest factor in developing Type 2 diabetes, other factors that play a role include the composition of the cell's lipid membranes, autoimmune factors, and even the health of one's intestinal flora.

more depending on how long it has taken to detect an increased fasting glucose. Despite much higher fasting and postprandial insulin levels, the body can no longer keep the fasting glucose in the 70 to 80 mg/dL range and the fasting glucose begins to move into the abnormal range.

Even though the body's glucose metabolism has been breaking down and has been severely compromised for as long as a decade or two, the fasting glucose level, which is the last thing to "break," is only just now beginning to leave the normal range. Sadly, it's the fasting glucose level that most physicians rely upon when diagnosing a patient as a Type 2 diabetic.

Why Looking at Only the Fasting Glucose Level Is Not Enough

Many of the clinical guidelines in use today encourage a physician to use fasting glucose as the sole indicator of one's diabetic health. Seeing a fasting glucose level within the laboratory "normal" range, both patient and physician are satisfied that the patient is at low risk of Type 2 diabetes.

Now that you know more about how diabetes progresses, you can see that gauging the risk of Type 2 diabetes solely on fasting glucose is terribly ineffective. An abnormal fasting glucose is typically the *last* commonly used indicator to show the presence of diabetes. In fact, by the time your fasting glucose is no longer in the normal range, *you are already diabetic.*

The message here is this: Use fasting glucose as one of the many tools to diagnose your risk of diabetes, but not as the sole measure of your diabetes risk, because by the time your fasting glucose "breaks," your body's glucose metabolism is probably irreparably degraded.

Damage from Elevated Glucose versus Damage from Elevated Insulin

This chapter has discussed the damaging effects of elevated glucose levels and elevated insulin levels, almost as though they're interchangeable. But that's not the case.

While elevated glucose and elevated insulin are both harmful, I believe elevated glucose levels are far more damaging than elevated insulin levels.

I say this because comparing insulin-dependent Type 1 diabetics and insulin-dependent Type 2 diabetics reveals that if their glucose levels are poorly controlled, both groups experience the same severe diabetes complications, despite the fact that Type 1 diabetics typically take much less insulin than insulin-dependent Type 2 diabetics require. (Recall that a Type 1 diabetic is someone whose body can make virtually no insulin whatsoever.)

The American Diabetes Association Guidelines and You

The American Diabetes Association (ADA) guidelines will most likely indicate that you are fine—right up until the moment that you are an irreparably damaged diabetic. Let's take a look at the ADA's guidelines for diagnosing diabetes and see why they and your doctor, if he or she uses the ADA guidelines, wait far too long before diagnosing someone as a diabetic.

The term *diabetic* means that our ability to metabolize glucose is compromised. The goal is to recognize as early as possible that we are diabetic, so that we can avoid ever having diabetic complications or needing to take insulin.

Testing for Diabetes

In the preceding section, we saw that our postprandial glucose response is typically the first indicator that something is wrong with glucose metabolism, typically becoming abnormal years or decades before the fasting glucose level climbs out of range. Yet the ADA says that for testing for diabetes in patients without symptoms (i.e., testing to detect Type 2 diabetes and assess risk for future diabetes), "either A1C, FPG [fasting glucose], or OGTT [oral glucose tolerance test] are appropriate."[1]

---

1. American Diabetes Association, "Standards of Medical Care in Diabetes—2010"

If you are one of the fortunate people whose physician decides that an oral glucose tolerance test is the way to go, then your diabetes may be detected a decade or more before the person whose physician uses the cheaper fasting glucose to gauge diabetes risk. And with insurance companies increasingly concerned about saving money, do you think they will be quick to pay for an oral glucose tolerance test when the ADA advises that the cheaper fasting glucose test is equally valid?

The ADA, Fasting Glucose, and A1C

As shown in the table below, the American Diabetes Association's *Standards of Medical Care in Diabetes–2010* guidelines uses A1C and fasting glucose values to classify people as *normal*, *at risk*, or *diabetic*.

	Normal	**At Risk**	**Diabetic**
A1C	< 5.7%	5.7–6.4%	> 6.4%
Fasting Glucose	<100 mg/dL	100–125 mg/dL	> 125 mg/dL

In my opinion, these guidelines are misguided at best and dangerous at worst.

If you look on the ADA website (and most other sites that discuss using an A1C value to derive an average glucose level), they will provide a single average glucose level for a given A1C value, as though the two correlate perfectly. As with most statistical correlations, however, showing a single glucose value for a given A1C value does not take into account the error inherent in the conversion.

If we consider the statistical margin of error[1] in the A1C to average glucose estimate (see *Limitations to the A1C Test* on page 68), the following table shows the average glucose ranges that the above

1. The statistical margin of error referred to here is known as the CI, or "confidence interval." The CI is the percentage of confidence that the value stated is due to the data and not due to chance. By saying "90–140 mg/dL with a 95% CI," the statistician is claiming to be 95% sure that the true value is somewhere in the stated range.

A1C values translate into, first as stated by the ADA and then when we take into account the true error in the calculations.[1]

A1C Value	Average Blood Glucose (as stated by ADA)	Average Blood Glucose (with 95% confidence)
5.6% (Normal)	114 mg/dL	90–140 mg/dL
6.0% (At risk)	126 mg/dL	100–152 mg/dL
6.5% (Diabetic)	140 mg/dL	112–169 mg/dL

Confidence interval notwithstanding, based upon the table you can see that the average glucose value associated even with the ADA's *normal* category (114 mg/dL) is alarmingly high. Looking at the 95% confidence interval, however, the fact that one can have *average* glucose values of 152 mg/dL and still be considered merely *at risk* for diabetes boggles the mind. According to Jenny Ruhl, in *Blood Sugar 101* and Dr. Richard Bernstein, in his book *Diabetes Solution*, blood glucose levels of 140 mg/dL are "toxic."

It's possible that an A1C of 6.0 actually represents an average blood glucose much closer to 150 mg/dL than it does to an ADA reported 126 mg/dL. If my average glucose is 150 mg/dL, it's a virtual certainty that my fasting glucose is around 100 mg/dL, if even that low. This means that I am routinely reaching postprandial blood sugars of 200 mg/dL or more, especially if I'm eating a high glycemic diet.

I hate to break it to you, but if this describes you, then you're not "at risk for diabetes," as the ADA states, you *already have* diabetes. And blood sugars this high are causing *significant damage* in your body every day.

This is one of the many reasons that the A1C fasting glucose tests are far inferior to checking your own postprandial glucose levels and seeing what your glucose values are during a typical day.

1. Range reported is for a 95% confidence interval. Nathan, DM, et al. Translating the A1C assay into estimated average glucose values. *Diabetes Care* 2008:31:1473–1478.

Pre-Diabetic and Other Labeling Nonsense

The most effective preventive health strategy is to use all the glucose metabolism tests, in their proper role and context, to create an accurate picture of your diabetes risk. Unfortunately, too many providers get tunnel vision on one of the tests and overlook the big picture.

If your doctor uses the ADA guidelines, as most clinicians do, for many years after you've become a diabetic, your doctor will still refer to you as a "pre-diabetic." The medical industry invented the term *pre-diabetic* in an attempt to give a label to those patients who were on the path to developing diabetes so that they could make appropriate lifestyle changes and minimize, or reverse, the course of the disease.

While this sounds like a great goal for the medical profession to set—helping people to recognize an impending disease in time to take action—it only works if the term *pre-diabetic* is used correctly, which it typically is not. A more accurate term might be *pre-insulin dependent diabetic*, because someone whom the ADA labels *pre-diabetic* probably doesn't yet require insulin, but such a person is likely already a diabetic and is suffering great harm from routinely elevated blood glucose levels.

The message here is very simple: *If you wait until your doctor tells you you're a diabetic before you take action to correct your diet and lifestyle, you have a much, much tougher battle to fight than if you take action sooner.*

OK! So I'm a Diabetic! What Now?

OK, you've bought a glucose meter, learned how to use it, and used up a box of 50 test strips obtaining a very solid picture of how a typical week's eating affects your blood glucose. And the picture isn't pretty: Even though your fasting glucose, the number that you and your doctor have been watching for years, is still in LabCorp's "normal range," your week of study has shown that you routinely reach blood glucose levels of 150 to 200 mg/dL within an hour or two after eating. Furthermore, this book, and perhaps the writings of Jenny Ruhl and Richard Bernstein, have convinced you that blood glucose levels above 110 mg/dL or so are harmful and 140 mg/dL and above are toxic.

Now what do you do?

First, take a deep breath and congratulate yourself. You probably now know more about diabetes than most people out there.

The second thing to remember is that we seem to have falsely equated *diabetic* with *insulin-dependent* in our thinking. *Diabetic* doesn't mean that your diabetes has progressed far enough that you are insulin-dependent—it just means that your ability to metabolize glucose is compromised.

The good news is that no matter where you are on the healthy versus at risk continuum or pre-diabetic versus diabetic continuum, there is still much that you can do to improve your condition, very possibly avoiding many of the complications that you would experience otherwise.

And even though this isn't really a book about diabetes, information about glucose control permeates this book. This is because elevated glucose and insulin are a principal component in virtually every malady that we face today, and most certainly a significant factor in cardiac health.

On page 129, you'll learn about daily strategies to help you reduce your insulin resistance (i.e., increase your insulin sensitivity), a key to preventing not only Type 2 diabetes but a host of accompanying maladies. More importantly, you'll learn even more about how your $20 glucose meter is your most cost-effective ally against obesity, diabetes, and heart disease, no matter who you are.

The Most Important Points from This Chapter

- The term *diabetic* means that the ability to metabolize glucose is compromised. It's possible to be a diabetic without the disease having yet progressed enough to require insulin.
- Most people who are diabetic don't know it.
- A fasting glucose test is a useful tool, but it should not be the primary test to see if you are diabetic.
- No matter what anyone's guidelines say, damage to your body occurs whenever your blood glucose level goes above 110 mg/dL and levels of 140 mg/dL and above are toxic.
- Insulin is one of the most powerful hormones in the body, responsible for a variety of roles, but primarily as a growth hormone that also forces the body to store fat in its fat cells.
- Insulin resistance is a significant factor not only in developing Type 2 diabetes but also in developing coronary artery disease.
- An inexpensive home glucose meter is a vital part of any weight loss plan as well as an effective tool in any preventive health effort.
- With the proper awareness, we can be given years, even decades, of warning. If we wait until traditional clinical guidelines say that we're a diabetic, we'll be fighting a much more difficult battle to keep the damaging effects of insulin resistance at bay.

If You Want to Take Action Immediately

- Buy a glucose meter and some test strips, learn how to use them, and start measuring your blood glucose when you first awaken in the morning and at one- and two-hour intervals after you finish each meal. A week of doing this will give you a very valuable picture of how your body metabolizes glucose, far more useful than any single test that your doctor would run (all for about $40). For some good sources of these supplies, see Appendix P.

- If your tests with the glucose meter show fasting glucose levels above 90 mg/dL and postprandial glucose levels above 110 mg/dL or 120 mg/dL, talk with your physician about ordering an official fasting glucose, a fasting insulin, and an A1C test. These will be useful in confirming what your home glucose readings have shown and also in establishing some baseline data that will be useful as you monitor your improvement. (I've talked about the usefulness of an oral glucose tolerance test, but if you have already amassed a considerable number of postprandial blood glucose readings showing such elevated glucose levels, I don't think an oral glucose tolerance test will tell you much more than you already know and may not be worth the assault on your body.) If your physician is unwilling to order these for you, consider doing so yourself from one of the companies online, as described in Appendix S.

4

Inflammation

According to Dr. Floyd Chilton, author of *Inflammation Nation*, nearly 50% of US residents suffer from an inflammatory disease. Nearly half of us! Inflammation plays a significant role in virtually every major disease, yet many people don't even know what *inflammatory disease* means.

Inflammation is the body's response to harmful stimuli. Like so many mechanisms in the body, inflammation is a double-edged sword. The right amount of inflammation, in the right circumstances, is vital whereas excessive or misdirected inflammation is harmful. An asthma attack, for example, is an excessive inflammatory response to an external factor, such as dust or pollen.

This chapter discusses the role of inflammation in the body, both good and bad, and the reasons that the inflammation process runs amok in so many of us. You'll also see references to *autoimmune disorders*. Autoimmune disorders are a type of inflammatory diseases where the body responds not to an external stimulus but instead attacks the body itself, mistakenly interpreting normal body tissues as invaders. Autoimmune disorders are at the heart of a variety of maladies, including Type 1 diabetes, rheumatoid arthritis, and thyroid disease.

The Role of Inflammation

Looking at the multi-billion dollar anti-inflammatory drug market, we might be tempted to view inflammation as being a bad thing that should never be allowed to happen. This, however, is far from true. Inflammation is a naturally occurring process that plays a vital role in our health and healing.

Inflammation: The Good

Why would a potentially damaging inflammatory response be a naturally occurring process? What beneficial purpose does inflammation play in the body? The term *inflammation* describes a series of events that occur when the body's immune system responds to an invader, like a virus or bacteria. When such an invader penetrates the body's defenses, the immune system responds, chemically signaling the immune system to the invader's presence so that various types of white blood cells can attack the invader.

Each type of white blood cell exhibits specific behavior and targets certain types of invaders. If you want to learn more about white blood cell behavior, research *neutrophils*, *macrophages*, *B lymphocytes*, and *T lymphocytes*. (I'm not sure which kind ate Donald Pleasence in the movie *Fantastic Voyage*, but that was my first introduction to white blood cells.)

Like any effective army, the attacking white blood cells have the ability to communicate and coordinate their actions. This communication occurs via chemical messages made from specialized forms of fatty acids. These chemical signals tell white blood cells where to go and also pave the way for their effective travel by dilating blood vessels so that the white blood cells can more quickly reach their destination. (Remember these fatty acid chemical messengers used by the white blood cells to coordinate their attack—they are key to understanding how the inflammatory process can run amok.) When these messaging systems work properly, white blood cells travel quickly to their destination, attack the correct invader with the properly measured response, cease attacking when the invader has been destroyed, and clean up the mess left behind from their efforts.

Inflammation: The Bad

Imagine, if you will, that instead of responding in a measured way to a bit of dust or pollen, the immune system reacts in full force, grossly over-functioning in relation to the magnitude of the minor threat. This sort of over functioning might manifest itself as an asthma attack or an allergic reaction, producing a response that's far more harmful and disruptive than the invader that was initially targeted.

Similarly, the inflammation response might be of the proper magnitude but might continue far longer than the situation demands. This type of over-functioning inflammation leads to a chronic, as opposed to acute, inflammatory response and leads to diseases like psoriasis, rosacea, or Crohn's disease, where the body's immune system continues a low-level assault on healthy tissues for prolonged periods.

Whether they are acute or chronic, inflammatory diseases share the common theme of the body's own immune system functioning beyond its necessary role, producing excessive inflammation and causing further damage to the structures of the body.

Autoimmune Disorders

A specific type of inflammatory disorder, known as an *autoimmune disorder*, doesn't need an external invader to trigger an overactive response. *Autoimmunity* means that the body's immune system mistakes normal, healthy structures in the body for invaders and attacks them. Examples of autoimmune diseases include rheumatoid arthritis (where the body attacks its own joints), scleroderma (skin hardening due to excessive collagen production), and lupus. Autoimmune disorders are especially insidious because once an autoimmune disorder manifests itself, the immune system continues attacking undeserving parts of the body constantly and without external provocation.

While nobody knows with absolute certainty what causes autoimmune disorders, the evidence is becoming clear that a major contribution to autoimmune disease is the immune system confusing the body's structures with external substances that are chemically similar. For example, human and animal studies have identified a number of environmental and dietary substances that increase the incidence of the autoimmune disease lupus, in which the body attacks various structures, including chromosomal proteins and DNA, as though they were foreign invaders.[1] A study in a heavily industrialized area of Georgia shows that residents who were exposed to a higher level of airborne industrial pollutants were nine times more likely to develop lupus.[2]

Evidence that dietary proteins play a role in rheumatoid arthritis is provided by studies that placed participants on a strict diet that minimized exposure to certain proteins and showed a reduction in arthritis symptoms.[3] While factors causing inflammation will almost certainly vary from person to person, this study gives credibility to the argument that diet is a worthy place to begin searching for specific inflammatory triggers.

What research is beginning to show is that prolonged exposure to substances that *mimic* structures and compounds native to the human body can cause the immune system to be confused, especially when immune systems are weakened by such things as overwork, stress, poor diet, or age.

Because such exposures can happen over a long period of time and because our sensitivity is often a result of a unique combination of dietary and environmental factors, it can be very difficult to link specific triggers with specific inflammatory diseases, forcing us and our physicians to resort to trial and error to identify the triggers. Nonetheless, it seems obvious that diet, environmental contaminants, and even certain medications can be a factor. The section *Specific Causes of Excessive Inflammation* on page 89 discusses some suspected inflammatory triggers.

---

1. Malathion, the insecticide, has been shown to cause lupus in genetically susceptible rodents. While not conclusive proof that it will do so in humans, it certainly causes concern.

2. Kardestuncer T, Franklin H. Systemic lupus erythematosus in relation to environmental pollution: an investigation in an African-American community in North Georgia. *Archives of Environmental Health*, 1997;52(2):85–90.

3. Kjeldsen-Kragh J, et al. Controlled trial of fasting and one-year vegetarian diet in rheumatoid arthritis. *Lancet* 1991;338(8772):899–902.

Common Examples of Inflammatory and Autoimmune Diseases

There are many different inflammatory and autoimmune diseases. Common examples include the following:

- **Celiac disease (gluten intolerance)**—Proteins in glutens mimic a number of naturally occurring proteins in the body, causing inflammation, both chronic and acute. Gluten intolerance is so common today that the evils of grains could fill a chapter of their very own. See page 123 for more information about grains and their dangers.
- **Type 1 diabetes**—Due to an autoimmune attack on the insulin-producing cells of the pancreas, a person suddenly loses the ability to produce insulin. While nobody knows exactly why such an attack occurs, many speculate that a combination of genetic susceptibility and external inflammatory triggers is responsible.
- **Asthma**—This is a chronic inflammation of the airways, most commonly caused by an allergic reaction to inhaled or ingested substances. Numerous studies have identified inflammatory omega-6 fatty acids in vegetable oils as a trigger for asthma development.
- **Leaky gut**—Leaky gut describes a less than effective bond between adjacent cells in the intestinal walls, which causes toxins and undigested proteins to enter the bloodstream, producing further inflammatory response. What causes this increase in intestinal permeability? Wheat does, and so do elevated glucose levels.
- **Thyroid disorders**—The thyroid is extremely susceptible to autoimmune attack, typically producing hypothyroidism (reduced thyroid function).

- **Multiple sclerosis**—MS causes the immune system to attack the central nervous system. This is believed to be caused by a combination of genetic susceptibility and exposure to certain wheat and dairy products.[1]
- **Crohn's disease/Ulcerative colitis**—Collectively known as *irritable bowel disease*, these maladies are caused by the immune system attacking the intestines. Evidence points to wheat gluten sensitivity as a significant factor in irritable bowel disease.[2]
- **Coronary artery disease**—My favorite topic! Keep reading.

Inflammation and Coronary Artery Disease

While my interest in preventive health focused initially on coronary artery disease, moving from heart disease to inflammation was a very short leap. This is because inflammation causes arterial damage and produces areas of the artery that are infiltrated by small, opportunistic LDL particles and then become further inflamed. This leads to an increased response by the immune system, resulting in a crusty, unstable plaque formation that is in constant danger of rupturing and causing a heart attack. Though the mechanism of action can be complex, there's no longer any doubt that inflammation plays a central role in coronary artery disease.

As two researchers state:

> ...atherosclerosis, the main cause of CAD [coronary artery disease], is an inflammatory disease in which immune mechanisms interact with metabolic risk factors to initiate, propagate, and activate lesions in the arterial tree.[3]

---

1. Cordain, L. Cereal grains: Humanity's double-edged sword: Evolutionary aspects of nutrition and health. Diet, exercise, genetics and chronic disease. *World Review of Nutrition and Dietetics.* 1999; 84: 19–73.

2. Cordain, L. Cereal grains: Humanity's double-edged sword: Evolutionary aspects of nutrition and health. Diet, exercise, genetics and chronic disease. *World Review of Nutrition and Dietetics.* 1999; 84: 19–73.

3. Hansson, GK. Mechanisms of disease: Inflammation, atherosclerosis, and coronary artery disease. *New England Journal of Medicine* 2005;352:1685–1695.

> The appreciation that inflammation is a fundamentally important component of atherosclerotic lesion initiation and progression has fundamentally altered our view of the [step-by-step development] of atherosclerosis.[1]

For more information on inflammation's role in causing coronary artery disease, see Chapter 5.

Specific Causes of Excessive Inflammation

Identifying specific causes of inflammation can be difficult. Food sensitivities, for example, can take 36 hours or longer to induce inflammatory symptoms, making it nearly impossible to correlate inflammation with a trigger food. Some foods, like wheat, can cause such a consistent low level of inflammation that the symptoms never appear to be acute, instead lingering below the level of our attention for decades until they finally manifest as inflammatory bowel diseases like Crohn's disease and ulcerative colitis.

Other inflammatory factors, environmental contaminants, for example, can require months or years of exposure before the immune system becomes sensitive and starts overreacting.

Even when inflammation executes properly by destroying harmful invaders and then subsiding, some collateral damage may occur. If we have a normal inflammation response, this collateral damage is minimal and is cleared away by the body's normal healing process. However, a significant danger with excessive inflammation is the continuously occurring damage that incessantly taxes the body's repair processes. Additionally, the damage caused by the inflammation is itself a source of further inflammation as the immune system over-responds to the damage that it's causing the body, producing a "runaway train" effect where factors that once caused no immune response now do so.

---

1. Ballantyne, CM, ed. *Clinical lipidology: A companion to Braunwald's heart disease.* New York, NY: Saunders, 2009.

Environmental Causes of Inflammation

Any chemical or particulate that we encounter, even at low levels, can be an environmental cause of inflammation. Common sources include air fresheners, household cleaners, synthetic fibers (e.g., dust and fibers from carpets and furniture), airborne heavy metals and chemicals, and virtually any chemical that we're exposed to on a regular basis.

While this chapter focuses primarily on dietary sources of inflammation, plenty of opportunities are available to significantly reduce the levels of environmental inflammatory triggers that we expose ourselves to every day. Consider the cleaning products you use at home. Do you really need to use an aerosol cleaner containing a frightening array of toxic chemicals when a simple spray bottle with white vinegar and water would do just fine? Consider the air freshener that you spray (or plug into an electrical outlet). They're far more than a fresh scent—they're an array of chemical irritants that you're continually breathing into your body.

Do you need to expose your skin and your lungs to a furniture polish made from "naphtha, petroleum, light alkylate; dimethicone; butane; isobutane; and propane"[1] when an olive oil, linseed oil, lemon juice, and water mixture will work just as well?[2]

Obviously, it's not possible to remove every single cause of inflammation from our environment, but taking simple steps like replacing chemical-laden household chemicals with safer (and often cheaper!) homemade alternatives and minimizing our exposure to chemical contaminants can go a long way toward helping to reduce inflammation in our bodies. Even the simple step of purchasing an air purifier that helps remove airborne contaminants can help calm an overexcited immune system. When it comes to reducing inflammation, every little bit helps.

---

1. Pledge® Clean and Dust Furniture Polish Material Safety Data Sheet, 2009, SC Johnson Co.

2. Berthold-Bond, A. *Clean and green: The complete guide to nontoxic and environmentally safe housekeeping.* Woodstock, NY: Ceres Press, 1994.

Age-Related Causes of Inflammation

There's no escaping it: As we age, our immune system weakens, becoming less effective and more easily confused, leading to a natural increase in inflammation. The best way to combat the age-related decline in our immune system's effectiveness is to maintain a lifestyle that minimizes inflammation and promotes immune system health, a subject of much research that could easily fill its own book. Suffice it to say that you can maximize your immune system's effectiveness by maintaining a proper diet, taking the necessary nutritional supplements, sleeping adequately, minimizing stress, minimizing alcohol intake, and avoiding tobacco. Giving your immune system less to do, by avoiding infections, will also help avoid excessive inflammation.

Dietary Causes of Inflammation

As inflammatory as environments can be, for most people, diet is the single largest cause of inflammation. Recall that inflammatory responses are initiated by fatty acid messengers that are released at the site of inflammation and signal to the body to commence a proper inflammatory response. These messengers (primarily leukotrienes and protaglandins) are manufactured by the body using an omega-6 fatty acid called arachidonic acid (AA). Because AA is the principal component of these inflammation chemical messengers, AA is an essential fatty acid *but only in low levels.*

Think about it this way: The body uses AA in a very controlled way—as a signal to the immune system that says "create just the necessary amount of inflammation right here!" When the immune system detects this AA chemical messenger, it dutifully rounds up the necessary materials to begin the process of creating some localized inflammation, perhaps in response to pollen in the bronchial tubes or a bacterial invader or some other trigger. If the immune system is working properly, this is the only time inflammation happens.

Imagine a misguided person who wanted to induce inflammation in his body at will. How would he go about doing so? Simple—deposit that same omega-6 chemical messenger wherever he desired an inflammatory event, wait a moment or two, and voilà! inflammation appears! What if he does this to himself many times a day all over his body? What do you think will happen? At each place the immune system detects AA, it will say, "Yes, sir! Creating some inflammation right here! Just like you asked!"

We never have to worry about being this hypothetical masochist, though. We're following a heart-healthy diet that avoids unhealthy fats, so we don't have to worry about arachidonic acid from omega-6 consumption, right?

Hold that question for a moment and let's first talk about cell membranes.

A typical cell membrane is composed of a lipid bilayer, which is just what it sounds like: two layers of fatty acid molecules, sandwiched together to give cell membranes their much-needed strength. This bilayer also forms an effective barrier to foreign substances, through the use of embedded *receptors* that are designed to transfer only specific things into and out of the cell. The impermeable lipid layers and their receptors serve as gatekeepers to help ensure the health of a cell by transferring only what the cell needs, in the right amounts, into the cell and removing unwanted substances from within the cell. Virtually anything that the cell consumes or produces is transported this way, ensuring that only the proper substances ever reach the interior of the cell.

As with most structures of the body, the cell's lipid bilayer needs to be constantly maintained, which the body does by constantly replenishing the crucial fatty acids that comprise the cell membranes. What happens if a person eats a trivial amount of healthy omega-3 fatty acids and an abundance of unhealthy omega-6 fatty acid? Simple, the body does its best with what you give it and will use the omega-6 fatty acids instead.

What this means is that in addition to their role in promoting inflammatory chemical messengers, omega-6 fatty acids become incorporated into *virtually every cell in your body.*

The problem with this is that omega-3 fatty acids are designed to be strong yet flexible, allowing the cell membrane to bend and flex properly as the body's demands dictate. An example would be the walls of arterial vessels, which need to be strong yet flexible to handle the constantly changing pressure of blood flow. In contrast, omega-6 fatty acids form brittle, inflexible structures that do not flex and that crack easily under pressure.

Imagine what happens if the strong, flexible omega-3 fatty acids in your cell membranes are replaced with brittle, easily fractured omega-6 fatty acids. Instead of bending and flexing, expanding and contracting, the cells and arteries become more easily damaged, forming cracks and fissures that serve as homes for unfavorable lipid particles and causing even more inflammation.[1]

Once again, that's okay, though. We're following a heart-healthy diet that avoids fat, so we don't have to worry about arachidonic acid from omega-6 consumption, right?

I wish it were so.

The horrible truth is that the AA-containing omega-6 fatty acids aren't in the fats that the "experts" are telling you to *avoid*. They're in many of the fats that the so-called experts are telling you to eat as part of a heart-healthy diet!

I'll say it again: The single biggest source of highly inflammatory, heart disease-inducing omega-6 fatty acids are the "heart-healthy" oils that we are being told to eat as part of a heart-healthy diet.

We'll talk later about optimizing omega-3 and omega-6 intake, but I'll give you a hint now: the ideal omega-6 fatty acid intake is in the range of three grams to six grams in an *entire day*.[2] Now take a look

---

1. In *The Essential Omega-3 Diet*, Evelyn Tribole quotes the NIH's *essential fats education* program as saying that excessive omega-6 fats in the diet trigger a rise in heart attacks, blood clots, arthritis, asthma, menstrual cramps, headaches, and tumor metastases.

2. This assumes that a person is consuming the correct amount of healthy omega-3 fatty acids, which very few people do.

at this table that shows the amount of omega-6 fatty acids in some foods that are commonly believed to be good for us.

"Healthy" Oils	Omega-6 per Tablespoon
Promise brand heart-healthy spread	3.2 grams
Smart Balance brand buttery spread	2.3 grams
Soybean oil-laden imitation mayonnaise	3.4 grams
Cottonseed oil	7 grams
Corn oil	7 grams
Grapeseed oil	9.5 grams
Safflower oil	10 grams
Sesame oil	5.6 grams
Soybean oil	7 grams

Now let's compare the insanely high omega-6 levels in the "heart-healthy" items above to some more favorable oils:

Truly Healthy Oils	Omega-6 per Tablespoon
Coconut oil	0.24 grams
Palm kernel oil	0.22 grams
Olive oil	1.32 grams

If the ideal amount of omega-6 fatty acid intake is somewhere around three to six grams in a day, how much omega-6 does the typical person eat? According to Evelyn Tribole, author of *The Essential Omega-3 Diet*, the typical American diet includes *10 to 20 times* the recommended maximum amount of omega-6 fatty acids.

Ten to twenty times? How is this possible?

It's simple: Pick up nearly any food item and take a look at how common omega-6 oils are. They're in virtually everything we eat. Wander through the grocery store (or even your own pantry) and look at how many foods contain soybean oil, cottonseed oil, corn oil, safflower oil, or any of the many other omega-6-laden oils commonly in use today. They're nearly unavoidable.

The reason they're so common is very simple: They're cheap to produce, which makes them very profitable to sell. If you're curious, read or watch Dr. Mary Enig's *Oiling of America* to learn about economic factors driving "heart-healthy" industrial oil products—products that are a significant cause of heart disease.

By the way, you'll note the presence of coconut oil in the table of favorable oils. Coconut oil is one of the most baselessly maligned oils out there. Over half of the fat in coconut oil is lauric acid, a medium-chain fatty acid that has been shown in countless studies to have significant health benefits.

Seeing how common these inflammation promoters are, it's no wonder why so many people have rheumatoid arthritis, allergies, headaches, and a host of other inflammatory and autoimmune disorders. Excessive omega-6 intake is even more likely among those who subscribe to the "low-fat is good" thinking because virtually all of the fat a person on such a diet eats is "heart-healthy" vegetable oil-based fats.

One of the frustrating things about omega-6 fatty acids is that food packages rarely disclose the presence of omega-6 fatty acids, making it difficult to determine just how much omega-6 fatty acid we're eating in a day. To address this, I've turned to books such as *The Ultimate Omega-3 Diet* to identify how much omega-6 is present in everything I eat. Minimizing or avoiding processed foods makes this task easier by allowing me to focus on 20 or 30 naturally occurring foods instead of countless thousands of processed ones.

What I find more frightening about inflammation is the startling evidence that it's not just adults who are suffering from inflammatory disorders at an alarming rate, but that our children are too. We need only look around to see countless "peanut-free" school zones and at all the asthmatic children to realize that allergies and other autoimmune diseases are on a dramatic rise among children and even infants, who certainly haven't had time to build up chronic autoimmune disorders from decades of environmental exposure and "heart-healthy" omega-6 fatty acids. What's happening with the children? How can a 3- or 4-year-old have an immune system that is so precarious as to cascade into anaphylactic shock over a single peanut or some pollen in the breeze?

Recent research gives us a clue as to why children and infants are experiencing increased rates of autoimmune diseases: Pregnant women who are suffering from inflammation and autoimmune disorders give birth to babies who are already suffering from inflammation and autoimmune disorders. Combine this with a common childhood diet laden with highly inflammatory wheat and omega-6 fatty acids, and the results are peanut-free school zones and skyrocketing rates of childhood asthma.

Are you beginning to understand why heart disease has skyrocketed in the past 50 or 60 years? Do you think human genetics has radically changed in this timeframe or is it far more likely that a shift in our diet is responsible?

Combating Inflammation

The way to combat inflammation is to do everything possible to reduce the inflammation you already have and prevent further inflammation from occurring.

Yes, it seems obvious and it is pretty straightforward, but it requires a great deal of dedication and effort. It also requires that you give up the belief that because something has an American Heart Association logo on it, that it must be good for you.

The chapter *Setting Goals* on page 129 is devoted to specific steps that promote optimal health, including dietary suggestions for combating inflammation.

The Most Important Points from This Chapter

- Inflammation is a naturally occurring process in the body, necessary for combating invading substances.
- When the immune system is working properly, inflammation occurs at the right intensity, is directed at the correct target for the correct duration, and causes minimal collateral damage.

- Taxing the immune system by poor health, nutrition, lack of rest, stress, age, and other factors reduces the immune system's effectiveness, leading to inaccurate immune response.
- Subjecting ourselves to inflammatory triggers, either environmental or dietary, dramatically increases the inflammation in the body.
- Inflammation promotes inflammation as the immune system continues to attack what it perceives as legitimate targets but which are actually just the collateral damage from previous inflammatory responses.
- So-called "heart-healthy" oils made from industrial oil, such as vegetable oil, soybean oil, cottonseed oil, and safflower oil, are one of the biggest dietary causes of inflammation in our lives.
- Signs of autoimmune and inflammatory attack include asthma, rheumatoid arthritis, migraines, dermatitis, irritable bowel syndrome, and countless others.
- Pregnant women who are suffering from inflammation give birth to infants who are combating inflammation and autoimmune disorders, giving rise to asthma, allergies, and other infant and childhood autoimmune disorders that are prevalent today.

If You Want to Take Action Immediately

- Immediately begin identifying and eliminating the dietary and environmental sources of inflammation in your life, as specified in this chapter and in the references cited.
- Consider having your C-reactive protein (hsCRP) tested to determine your current level of inflammation. I talk more about this inflammatory marker in *Inflammation Goals* on page 154.

5

What Really Causes Coronary Artery Disease?

If you've read this far, you probably have a very good idea of some of the biggest factors that lead to coronary artery disease. While some factors are genetic, I believe the biggest controllable factors in heart disease are lipids, glucose metabolism, and inflammation. Often thrown into the mix are hypothyroidism and hormone imbalances, far too common in people over 40.

THE FORMATION OF PLAQUE

This chapter is not going to be a scientific treatise on the biochemistry of plaque formation. That subject is far too tedious, complex, and uncertain. I'm not a lipidologist nor am I a cardiologist. I'm just an everyday person trying to better understand plaque formation—a topic that has been simplified far too much. The biggest message here is that plaque formation is not caused by "saturated fat that you eat clogging your arteries." That dangerously simplistic message has survived far too long and has harmed far too many people by propelling the low-fat, high-grain madness that we've all endured.

People tend to think of plaque as a plug that clogs arteries, but due to the nature of plaque deposition within the arteries, I imagine plaque as something more like a scab than a plug. Plaque forms when very small, oxidized lipid particles lodge in small cracks in the arterial walls. The sticky, foamy goo that results continues to oxidize and invokes a response (sometimes an over-response) from the body's immune system, causing a scab-like growth that's partially embedded within the arterial wall, thickening the wall and making its once pliable, flexible nature crusty and brittle.

As the plaque continues to build up, the body's immune system continues to respond, sending white blood cells to the site to attack the bacteria that's growing within the plaque goo (bacteria that can be partially caused by harmful mouth bacteria that migrates into the bloodstream). These bacteria-laden particles of goo continue to oxidize (their oxidation enabled by lack of vitamin E and other antioxidants in the body), causing even more of an inflammatory response.

Meanwhile, elevated insulin levels cause the arterial walls to thicken even further, while high levels of glucose cause further arterial damage. High levels of omega-6 fatty acids in the diet further promote systemic inflammation and ensure that whatever repair is attempted on the arterial walls results in brittle, inflexible fatty acids being inserted at the repair site.

Highly oxidized saturated fats, bonded with glucose molecules join the party in the form of advanced glycated end products (AGEs), which are sticky, highly reactive particles that lodge in the arterial cracks, adding to the scab-like plaque that's growing there.

If we have high levels of genetically influenced Lp(a), the Lp(a) particles combine with homocysteine to further enhance the foamy, heavily oxidized, sticky, crusty plaque goo.

The liver, meanwhile, is busy creating LDL to help repair cellular damage because that's one of LDL's major functions. Due to hypothyroidism, high glucose levels, and excessive triglycerides brought on by a high carbohydrate diet[1] (primarily wheat but also including fructose, which is low glycemic but causes the liver to spew out triglycerides), the liver doesn't produce fluffy, helpful LDL particles. Instead, it produces small, dense LDL particles that oxidize more readily and serve as a source for additional plaque formation.

Meanwhile, the lack of dietary potassium and magnesium (very common today), coupled with more "heart-healthy" omega-6-laden vegetable oils, continues to drive blood pressure upward,[2] further damaging the arteries and constantly hammering on the scab-like plaque with increased pressure waves each time the heart beats.

More oxidation happens as the plaque continues to grow and the arterial wall thickens further with embedded plaque. Soon the wall will have thickened as much as it can and the plaque will begin growing inward.

If the plaque has enough time, the inward growth will form a restriction, producing detectable cardiac symptoms like shortness of breath or angina or abnormalities on a stress test. If the plaque hasn't formed a detectable obstruction, the plaque will continue to grow silently within the arterial wall, being hammered by pulsating pressure waves from high blood pressure.

More carbohydrates from a "heart-healthy" high-grain meal, coupled with some inflammatory "heart-healthy" vegetable oils, and the plaque continues to grow until finally its scab-like surface cracks, oozing foamy, bacteria-laden goo into the bloodstream.

---

1. In a small percentage of people, lipid metabolism is broken and they do produce unfavorable lipid particles in response to an excessive saturated fat intake. This is the rare exception rather than the rule, however.

2. But don't be so quick to blame salt for your high blood pressure: Moyer, MW. It's time to end the war on salt, *Scientific American*, July 8, 2011, p. 107.

The body responds predictably to the invader, forming a blood clot, which travels to a point of natural or plaque-induced narrowing and lodges there. Slight discomfort becomes intense pain and someone's life changes forever.

As you can see, there are many players in the drama of plaque formation. While genetics certainly plays a role, most notably in the form of Lp(a), many of the culprits in plaque formation are promoted by lifestyle decisions that:

- Cause the liver to produce small, dense LDL.
- Elevate glucose and insulin levels.
- Induce inflammation to produce cracks and fissures that act as breeding grounds for plaque formation.
- Produce Advanced Glycated End Products (AGEs) that form a basis for plaque.
- Form oxidizing agents in the body that cause the small dense, LDL to become even more heart-disease promoting.
- Cause thyroid dysfunction (frequently brought on by poor diet, especially excessive grains that promote autoimmune attack on the thyroid or insufficient iodine intake, a common occurrence).
- Disrupt hormones from processed food, toxins that leech from certain materials, and other environmental factors.
- Promote opportunistic bacteria from ineffective oral hygiene.
- Cause increased intestinal permeability, destroying gut health and promoting autoimmune responses.
- Erode cardiac conditioning through sedentary lifestyle.

How to Combat Plaque Formation

How do you combat plaque formation? That's simple. You attack every single one of the above causes, with as much vigor as you can muster, so that you can break the vicious cycle of plaque formation. You also test your lipids repeatedly so that you know if what you're doing is effective or not. And you monitor your plaque burden on a regular basis as the ultimate measure of your coronary artery disease.

Defining goals and making these important lifestyle changes are the focus of the second half of this book, "Part 2: Lifestyle Changes."

The Most Important Points from This Chapter

- There are many factors at play in plaque formation—it's nowhere near as simple as "eating saturated fat clogs your arteries."
- These factors provide many opportunities to break the cycle of plaque formation.
- It's not just the "blockage" that you have to worry about—any coronary plaque has the potential to cause a heart attack.

If You Want to Take Action Immediately

- Proceed to Part 2 of this book and begin making lifestyle changes.

Part 2: Lifestyle Changes

6

Dietary Truths, Half-Truths, and Fallacies

As you've learned in Part 1 of this book, effective preventive health requires that we:

- Control blood glucose levels
- Prevent inflammation from occurring
- Reduce existing inflammation
- Optimize lipid health (i.e., increase LDL particle size, reduce LDL particle count, increase HDL, and reduce triglycerides)

If these are the goals we choose for a healthy lifestyle, then any diet we choose must further these goals. Fortunately, as far as diet is concerned, these goals overlap a great deal and what benefits one goal typically helps many goals.

Unfortunately, however, deciding what a diet must do for us is the easy part. The difficulty lies in sorting through the maze of conflicting dietary advice to define exactly what an ideal diet is. While I've come to believe that there's no single ideal diet that will unilaterally bring optimum health to every human on the planet (we're just too varied for that to be possible), there are some fundamental dietary truths that benefit nearly everyone, some half-truths that get things somewhat right, and some fallacies that quite simply need to fade into obscurity for the good of everyone.

Dietary Truths

Vegetables are good for you.

Yes, they are. As long as you avoid the high-glycemic vegetables (for example, potatoes, corn, carrots, and beets), it's pretty hard to go wrong with veggies. I recommend that you try to buy vegetables directly from a local farmer who grows them, if possible, so that you have a better chance of getting foods that are what they're represented to be and are not genetically modified or riddled with insecticides. (For more about the harmful effects of genetically modified foods, see Appendix J.)

Include veggies of all types and colors with every meal and you'll be better for it. Even if you've completely given up grains, you won't have to worry about getting sufficient nutrients and fiber if you eat vegetables with every meal.

Processed, nitrate-laden meats are bad for you.

I'm going to agree with this one, too. Meats that are processed to lie on a shelf for months (or years) aren't something I want to eat.

And then there's bacon. When I have bacon, I try to have uncured, unprocessed bacon instead of processed bacon that's loaded with nitrates and nitrites. I admit that I'll have some cured bacon from time to time, but it's a rarity.

Overcooked, charred red meat is bad for you.

You're familiar by now with *advanced glycated end products* that result from cooking saturated fats at high temperatures. When I eat red meat, it's cooked rare or medium rare so that I minimize overcooked, oxidized saturated fats.

Processed foods are best avoided.

Processed food may be edible, but it isn't food to me. Paraphrasing Floyd H. Chilton, author of *Inflammation Nation*, food is something that looks like it did when it was growing or being raised. It's very rare that I encounter a processed food that is without some harmful ingredient like wheat, sugar, vegetable oil, or one of the other components that may be "generally recognized as safe" but certainly aren't healthy to eat. The safest thing to do with processed food is to leave it on the grocery store shelf where it belongs.

It's important to drink plenty of water.

Six glasses a day? Eight? I don't know what the magic number is, but I do believe that most people don't drink enough clean, pure water. Buy a good reverse osmosis filtration system for your home and drink plenty of water.

GBHs and GMOs are harmful.

True. GBHs are "glyphosate-based herbicides," which are poisons that are sprayed on genetically modified plants (GMOs, sometimes called "Roundup-ready" because the product Roundup is the most commonly known glyphosate-based herbicide). Unfortunately, tests are showing these herbicides and the GMOs are harmful to humans. See Appendix J for more information.

DIETARY HALF-TRUTHS

Saturated fat is bad for you.

Saturated fat has long been the whipping boy of the nutritional debate. It's so easy and convenient to create an image of "artery-clogging saturated fat" and drive that point home to sell enormously profitable low-fat and grain-based products that it's no wonder saturated fat has taken it on the chin.

It's sad, really, because saturated fat and, by inclusion, cholesterol, has been a principal component of the human diet since the beginning of recorded history. I contend that blaming saturated fat for the global rise in heart disease is woefully misguided.

But there's no doubting that some evidence suggests that saturated fat can be a factor in cardiac health (and cancer). If what defenders of saturated fat say is true, that eating it is beneficial at best and benign at worst, what is it about the saturated fat we're eating today that's different from the saturated fat that humans have eaten since the beginning of recorded history?

For one thing, *oxidation*.

When our ancestors ate animal products, they didn't subject them to the harsh processing and cooking methods that we employ today. These processes cause the cholesterol in our food to become heavily oxidized, which changes the once beneficial substance into oxidized cholesterol, which is highly reactive and contributes to the formation of cardiac plaque.[1]

How is the cholesterol we're eating becoming oxidized? In most any way that involves high temperatures and processing. For example:

Spray Drying — Spray drying is a process where a liquid is sprayed into a heated column that rapidly evaporates the liquid component of the mixture, leaving the solid behind to be collected. Violently agitating the finely ground particles in the extreme temperatures of the spray dryer causes them to be highly oxidized and can radically alter the properties of the material.

I was surprised to learn that countless food products are spray dried during their processing, including foods that I would never have suspected. For example, because eggs are so easily damaged and are so perishable, most baked goods produced by large manufacturing companies use spray-dried eggs. Spray-drying eggs reduces them to a very fine powder and exposes them to temperatures as high as 392° F (200° C).[2] (Of course, more than just spray-dried eggs make commercially manufactured baked goods an unfavorable dietary choice.)

Milk is another commonly spray-dried product, even organic milk. The organic milk you buy at the grocery store might have been obtained from a dairy cow in another country, spray dried, shipped to the United States as a fine, highly oxidized powder, and mixed with water to turn it back into "milk" for sale at your grocery store. Despite such extreme processing, this milk can still be labeled "organic." I'll leave it to you to decide how the result of this high-temperature spray drying process compares to fresh, organic milk.

Spray-dried, powdered milk is also routinely added to 1% and 2% milk to give it body, ensuring that such products are a potent source of oxidized cholesterol.

Protein powders are also frequently manufactured using spray drying, altering not only the structure of the proteins in the pow-

---

1. Addis P, Food and Nutrition News, March/April 1990, 62: (2):7–10.

2. GEA Process Engineering, Inc. http://www.niroinc.com/drying_dairy_food/spray_drying_pretreatment_eggs.asp

der but also oxidizing any cholesterol that's in the product. Not all protein powders contain cholesterol and not all of those are spray dried, but enough are that I try to seek out the ones that are not. This means that I assume any protein powder is spray dried at high temperature unless the manufacturer states otherwise.[1]

High-Temperature Cooking — According to many experts, we are cooking our cholesterol-rich foods at much higher temperatures than was common in the past. High temperature grilling and frying produce much higher levels of oxidized cholesterol than basting or slow roasting.

In addition to oxidation, there's another factor that alters the beneficial and benign saturated fat to produce a harmful dietary component: *glycation*.

As discussed previously, glycation of saturated fats is the process of saturated fats bonding to sugar (glucose) in the body, producing highly reactive, damaging, compounds called advanced glycated end products (AGEs).

Because AGEs are most commonly caused by elevated blood glucose levels, you'll see that AGEs are not an indictment on saturated fats but rather they're testament to the evils of elevated glucose levels and the carbohydrate-laden diets that cause them.

Because AGE formation is a product of two factors, glucose and saturated fats, either one can influence the levels of AGEs that form in the body. The thinking goes something like this: Heavily oxidizing the saturated fats when cooking them at extremely high temperatures makes fats more reactive and therefore more likely to bond with glucose, no matter the glucose level in the body. On the other hand, if one eats gently cooked, non-oxidized saturated fats but has a very high glucose level in the body, the person is just boosting the other side of the fat/glucose reaction by increasing the amount of glucose available.

---

1. A valid question is this: For foods other than protein powders, how do I know that something has been spray dried? There's no easy answer. Much about food processing is not widely divulged to the buying public. Issues like these motivate me to avoid processed foods altogether. I won't say I never eat processed foods any more, but it's exceedingly rare.

In other words, you get a similar undesirable effect whether you make the saturated fat really reactive by overcooking it or whether you make the glucose in your body more reactive by increasing its concentration. The net effect of either is harmful AGEs. And, of course, the net effect of doing both—eating a continuous stream of heavily oxidized, overcooked saturated fats along with foods that continually elevate blood glucose levels— is far more damaging.

In the words of Dr. Davis, glucose plus saturated fats are "like gasoline on a fire." This interaction is undoubtedly the basis for the few studies out there that show saturated fats are harmful; these studies invariably involve people with very elevated glucose levels. Normalizing the results to negate glucose influence removes any link between saturated fats and heart disease. As a result, studies that purport to show damaging effects of saturated fats are really just proving the harmful effects of AGEs, which is a very different thing altogether.

Oxidation and glycation represent the bulk of what's wrong with saturated fat in our diet. Nearly every study I've read that indicts saturated fat as an unhealthy dietary component is really just revealing the effect of highly oxidized and/or glycated saturated fat, not the effect of beneficial, properly prepared saturated fat in the presence of normal blood glucose levels.

And finally, dyslipidemia, covered in Chapter 2, describes the small percentage of people whose metabolism is damaged, causing them to metabolize saturated fats unfavorably.

Fruits are good for you.

Well, sort of. And only in very small amounts. And much less so the newly bred varieties of fruits that contain far more sugar than the fruits of 30 or 40 years ago. And certainly not fruit juices, which are nothing more than liquid fructose.

A small amount of fruit, complete with the accompanying fiber, is probably okay for most people. The problem with fruits comes in the form of huge amounts of fruits, daily pitchers of fruit smoothies, and glasses of fruit juices. This is best avoided, largely because of the harmful effects of fructose.

For more information on the ills of fructose, see *Fructose is good for you.* on page 122.

Nuts are good for you.

The overwhelming majority of nuts are healthful. Some, however, are so laden with omega-6 fatty acids that it's really tough to include a significant quantity of them in the diet and still maintain an optimum omega-6 and omega-3 balance. Examples of high omega-6 nuts include filberts and walnuts. Eat these in moderation to avoid having too much omega-6 fatty acid. And avoid the nut oils like walnut oil and the nut milks (e.g., almond milk) because they contain a huge amount of omega-6 fatty acids.[1]

Dietary "Truths" That Are Really Fallacies

We've looked at truths and half-truths. Now let's look at some fundamentally wrong dietary beliefs.

Eating fat is bad and should be avoided.

Most of Chapter 2, and the related content in Appendix A, shows that eating fat doesn't cause heart disease and, by extension, eating fat does not make you fat.

Fat is an absolutely vital component of a healthy diet. Most of the vital structures in your body, including the membranes of every cell, are made of fat. Your brain is about 60% fat. I think about the brain being 60% fat and cringe every time I see a parent give a small child, whose brain is still growing and developing, skim milk instead of whole milk (and I read about the health "experts" who are advocating putting children on statins). As Tom Naughton, producer of the documentary *Fat Head* says, we give our children skim milk and then wonder why they have poor concentration and ADD.

In adults, a low-fat diet paves the way for hormonal difficulties, cancer, dementia, and widespread cellular dysfunction as the body tries unsuccessfully to repair lipid-based structures without the proper fatty acid building materials to work with. This is especially

1. I speculate, but haven't yet verified, that naturally occurring omega-6 fatty acids from nuts are significantly less inflammatory than omega-6 fatty acids from processed industrial oils. As a result, I don't worry too much about occasionally eating something with a huge amount of almonds or other nuts (almond flour is a common replacement for wheat in lower-carb cooking).

problematic if the only fat you have when you're on your low-fat diet is "heart-healthy" omega-6-laden vegetable oils like safflower oil or soybean oil.

In fact, many physicians today recommend that a healthy diet obtains the *majority* of calories not from protein or carbohydrates but from *fat*.

Are some fats better than others? Of course. Just like some vegetables are better for you than others. The stigma of "artery-clogging saturated fat," however, is a baseless myth, propagated by bad science, politicians eager to make a name for themselves in the name of public good, and opportunistic food manufacturers. The depressing but historically fascinating study of how fiction was turned into an anti-fat campaign is perhaps best documented by science writer Gary Taubes.

Taubes' first book, *Good Calories, Bad Calories*, is a definitive tome on the hormonal effects of food and how politics and bad science demonized healthy foods that have served humankind for countless generations, while advocating higher-profit industrial oils and grains. *Good Calories, Bad Calories* is a must-read for anyone who wants to be informed about healthy eating and the public policies that have steered us away from the path of health and into the past half-century of obesity, diabetes, and heart disease.[1]

As Taubes and others have observed, the scientific method is often thwarted by human nature, most notably when scientists and public officials overlook contrary evidence because they just "know that their theory is right."

As Taubes says:

> A more insidious problem is that all involved—the researchers, the physicians, the public-health authorities, the health associations—commit themselves to a belief early in the evolution of the

1. In response to criticisms that the more than 500-page book was just too voluminous for the average reader to consume, Taubes wrote a more approachable version of *Good Calories, Bad Calories*, entitled *Why We Get Fat*, which is an elegant introduction into what's wrong with the horribly misguided advice to eat plenty of healthy grains and fruits and to avoid fats. If you're not up to *Good Calories, Bad Calories*, read *Why We Get Fat* instead. Then, if you're hungering for more, you can move on to *Good Calories, Bad Calories*.

> science, arguably at the stage at which they know the least about it, and then they become so invested in their belief that no amount of evidence to the contrary can convince them that they're wrong. As a result, when trials like the Women's Health Initiative find that eating less fat and less saturated fat has no beneficial effect [the Women's Health Initiative studied 49,000 middle-aged women for six years and found that a low-fat diet had no beneficial effect on heart disease, stroke, breast cancer colon cancer, or fat accumulation], the authorities don't respond by acknowledging that they have made an error all along. Doing so might make them (and us) question their credibility, as it should. Instead, they tell us that the study must have been flawed, and thus the results can be ignored.[1]

I've engaged a number of critics of Taubes who argue vehemently against his assertions, only to find that many of them haven't even read Taubes' books. Such uninformed critics are apparently responding in a knee-jerk fashion to hearing something that rocks their world: fat doesn't make you fat, calories don't count, and grains are unhealthy.

There are signs that the tide is turning. As I write this, Harvard University has issued a statement that we should give up the anti-fat hysteria and focus on the damaging effects of carbohydrates. Quoting Dr. Walter Willett, chairman of the Department of Nutrition at Harvard School of Public Health: "Fat is not the problem. If Americans could eliminate sugary beverages, potatoes, white bread, pasta, white rice and sugary snacks, we would wipe out almost all the problems we have with weight and diabetes and other metabolic diseases."[2]

Another fantastic introduction to the history of misguided dietary advice is comedian/satirist turned nutrition writer Tom Naughton's documentary *Fat Head* and his informative talk entitled *Big*

---

1. Taubes G. *Why We Get Fat*. New York, NY: Knopf, 2011.

2. As quoted in an article in *The Los Angeles Times*, December 20, 2010, "A Reversal on Carbs."

Fat Fiasco. Currently both are available at fathead-movie.com. *Fat Head* is a humorous documentary response to Morgan Spurlock's *Supersize Me*. In case you haven't seen *Supersize Me*, it is a "documentary" in which Spurlock eats countless hundreds of grams of carbohydrates per day for a month and becomes overweight and unhealthy. In response, he myopically ignores the role of his insanely high carbohydrate intake and blames his ill health on the fat in his diet, all with the pointed goal of painting McDonald's as a villain that has magically destroyed our ability to exercise free will. Naughton's documentary *Fat Head* and his similarly themed lecture *The Big Fat Fiasco* not only point out the blatant falsehoods and misrepresentations of *Super Size Me*, they also delve into the political maneuvering and scientific misrepresentation that brought about this entire "fat is bad" hysteria.

As you can frequently read on his fathead-movie.com blog, one of Naughton's favorite pastimes is exposing what he calls "bad science," in which researchers fall so thoroughly in love with their theories that they ignore or explain away clear evidence that their theory is wrong. I was saddened to learn that fraudulent or blatantly misleading research happens far more often than we might think. Dr. John Ioannidis is a biostatistician at the University of Ioannina in Greece and is considered one of the world's foremost experts on the credibility of medical research. He and his team have repeatedly shown that published research studies' conclusions (conclusions that doctors keep in mind when they make critical medical decisions) are misleading, exaggerated, or wrong as much as 90% of the time.[1]

A similar opinion is held by Dr. Marcia Angell, a former editor-in-chief of the New England Journal of Medicine. Dr. Angell stated, "It is simply no longer possible to believe much of the clinical research that is published, or to rely on the judgment of trusted physicians or authoritative medical guidelines. I take no pleasure in this conclusion, which I reached slowly and reluctantly over my two decades as an editor of The New England Journal of Medicine."[2]

---

1. Freedman, D. Lies, damned lies, and medical science, *The Atlantic*. November 2010.

2. Angell, M. Drug companies & doctors: A story of corruption. *New York Review of Books*, http://www.nybooks.com/January 15, 2009. http://www.nybooks.com/

It's known for certain that trans-fats (dubbed "Frankenfats" by biochemist Dr. Mary Enig), currently used in almost every available processed food, are highly damaging, inflammatory fats that never before existed. Unfortunately, many researchers lump highly inflammatory trans-fats and vegetable oils together with naturally occurring saturated fats in their human and animal studies and cite saturated fats as the culprit when writing their study conclusions.

Many studies on saturated fats also inadvertently study their effect in the presence of extremely high glucose levels, thereby distorting the results by the presence of AGEs and then blame saturated fats when they see an unfavorable outcome. AGEs are so damaging to the body that I believe anyone who has poorly controlled blood glucose levels should avoid saturated fats entirely. With glucose under control, however, it seems to be the exceedingly rare individual who has an unfavorable lipid response to saturated fats alone.

In the words of biochemist Richard Feinman, professor of biochemistry at Downstate Medical Center (SUNY) in New York, "Any deleterious effects of dietary fat have been measured in the presence of high carbohydrate. A high fat diet in the presence of high carbohydrate is different than a high fat diet in the presence of low carbohydrate."[1]

There's another reason for the widespread misunderstanding of fats in our diet: The subject of fats is very complex, with most medical reporters oversimplifying the subject. From my experience, most medical reports simply don't take the time to dig beyond the summary of a scientific paper, trusting at face value the conclusions the researchers present—research that Dr. Angell observes is not likely to be trustworthy.

1. Manninen A. Nutritional & metabolic aspects of carbohydrate restriction—An interview with Dr. Richard Feinman. *Nutrition and Metabolism Society.* May 2006. http://www.nmsociety.org/

Heart-healthy fats containing vegetable oils and soybean oils are healthy.

False. Reread *Dietary Causes of Inflammation* on page 91 and you'll see why vegetable oils are a primary dietary culprit in inflammation and heart disease.

Consuming fewer calories (along with burning more calories) will automatically cause a "calorie deficit" and will lead to a lower weight and less body fat.

If only it were this simple.

Yes, if we eat fewer calories than we burn, we'll lose weight and if we eat more calories than we burn, we'll gain weight. But the body is way too complex for this simplistic approach. I'll borrow an analogy from Tom Naughton's blog at *fathead-movie.com.*[1]

The "calories in/calories out" model is analogous to a checking account: If you put more money into an account than you spend, your account will have a positive growth and your account will grow (gain weight). If you spend more money from your checking account than you deposit, you'll have a negative growth and your checking account will shrink (lose weight). Ignoring for a moment that your checking account can go negative while your weight (presumably!) cannot, this is the model that most dieticians, nutritionists, and laypeople believe: to lose weight, simply eat fewer calories than you burn. As Naughton points out, this simplistic model assumes that deposits and withdrawals are independent, having no effect on each other.

In the human body, however, deposits and withdrawals are never independent. Returning to the bank analogy, cash deposits may be available immediately for spending whereas out-of-state checks may take several days to clear. Similarly, some foods you eat will be available for your body to metabolize immediately while some are more difficult to metabolize, depending on the hormone levels in your body. This is because elevated insulin levels lock fats into fat cells, making fat unavailable for metabolism, no matter how loudly the body is crying out for nourishment. In such a case, the calories consumed in the form of foods that elevate glucose and insulin

---

1. Naughton, T. "Fat accounts and the laws of fiscal dynamics." www.fathead-movie.com, January 25, 2011.

levels cause your body to respond very differently from those that do not elevate insulin levels.

In a bank deposit, a dollar is a dollar, quite unlike foods. Some foods, the gliadin proteins in wheat for example, stimulate appetite, making you even hungrier for having eaten them and prompting you to eat more while the exceedingly high glucose response from the wheat drives your insulin levels higher, further locking fat into your fat cells where it can't be metabolized. The result is eating without becoming sated, prompting more eating.

As insulin levels increase and the body becomes even less able to metabolize the high-energy fatty acids that are trapped in the fat cells, the body responds the only way it can to starving at the cellular level—it forces metabolism to slow down, dramatically reducing caloric demands. (As Naughton comments, this is like a bank having the authority to lower your thermostat or cancel elective expenses if it detects that your checking account is dangerously low—a far more complex, but accurate, analogy than simply "dollars in versus dollars out.")

This metabolic decline is even more pronounced when we respond to the weight gain by intentionally causing a calorie deficit in the hopes of losing weight, maybe even choosing "healthy whole grains," for their healthy fiber content, thus further increasing insulin levels in the body and further amplifying this cycle of insulin excess and cellular starvation. All the while, the cells in the body are screaming for nourishment and the gliadin proteins in the whole wheat products are inciting even more hunger. The result? Weight gain, elevated insulin, and misery for the person on a low-calorie diet.

The short answer here is that the body does obey the laws of thermodynamics—if a person eats fewer calories than she burns, she *will* lose weight. Achieving this goal, however, simply by counting calories and ignoring the hormonal effects of the foods we're eating is an exercise in absurdity and is perhaps the most ridiculous advice on dieting and health in the past 50 years.

A calorie is a nearly meaningless measure of a food's nutritional worth.

This wrongheaded thinking becomes entrenched through the efforts of such organizations as the American Dietetic Association (to be a "dietitian," one must have a bachelor's degree from a program accredited by the American Dietetic Association) who helps further the grain-based, "portion control," low-fat dogma that's gotten us all into this mess in the first place.[1]

In their continuing defense of this outdated model, many calories-in/calories-out advocates point out that a person eating 1,000 calories a day loses weight and a person eating 10,000 calories a day gains weight. This, they say, proves that it really is "all about calories."

Of course living at either of those extreme endpoints is going to have an effect. I can eat the most hormonally unfriendly foods out there and if I simply don't eat enough food, I'm going to lose weight. The weight will come from my muscles and organs before it comes from my fat cells (just like the obese hyperinsulinemic rats discussed above that starved to death without metabolizing any of their body fat), but I'll lose weight. And of course if I eat an unending torrent of hormonally optimal food, stuffing myself to bloated excess every single day, I'll gain weight, even without a massive insulin response.

In the middle of the bell curve, where we neither gorge ourselves nor starve ourselves insanely (and where optimal health resides), the hormonal influence of the food is far more relevant than the caloric count. What's more, an effective diet doesn't mean counting calories or being hungry all the time. Eating foods that promote a healthy hormone response (namely a healthy insulin response) is the primary requirement to a healthy diet. Do that and the body will settle down to a constant weight, *even with significant deviations in caloric intake.*[2]

In total, Taubes has written more than 700 pages on the subject and he says it much better than I do. Read *Why We Get Fat* and see why the calorie model of dieting is so sadly lacking. Taubes, by the way,

---

1. I have encountered some dieticians who recognize the dangers of low-fat diets, industrial oils, grains, and elevated glucose levels, but they're the minority.

2. I can attest that this is true for me, based upon a year's worth of daily food logs and monitoring my weight. With caloric intake that varies daily from zero to insanely high in a seeming random pattern, my weight has been within +/- a pound or so for over a year since I began eating foods that no longer promote a dramatic insulin response.

has a degree in physics from Harvard, so I'm pretty sure he understands the laws of thermodynamics, despite what his critics claim.

If Taubes' assertions are insufficient for you, however, I offer the work of Drs. Richard Feinman[1] and Eugene J. Fine, professors of biochemistry at the State University of New York Downstate Medical Center and Department of Nuclear Medicine, Jacobi Medical Center, Bronx, respectively:

> A review of simple thermodynamic principles shows that weight change on isocaloric diets is not expected to be independent of path (metabolism of macronutrients) and indeed such a general principle would be a violation of the second law. Homeostatic mechanisms are able to insure that, a good deal of the time, weight does not fluctuate much with changes in diet—this might be said to be the true "miraculous metabolic effect"—but it is subject to many exceptions. The idea that this is theoretically required in all cases is mistakenly based on equilibrium, reversible conditions that do not hold for living organisms and an insufficient appreciation of the second law. The second law of thermodynamics says that variation of efficiency for different metabolic pathways is to be expected. *Thus, ironically the dictum that a "calorie is a calorie" violates the second law of thermodynamics, as a matter of principle* [emphasis mine].[2]

Translated, this means that the argument for "a calorie is a calorie" is quite simply balderdash.

If this wasn't indictment enough, the authors conclude their paper by saying, "Attacking the obesity epidemic will involve giving up many old ideas that have not been productive. 'A calorie is a calorie' might be a good place to start."

---

1. He refers to himself as "Richard Feinman—The Other," for you nanotechnology geeks out there.

2. "Feinman, RD, Fine, EJ. "A calorie is a calorie" violates the second law of thermodynamics. *Nutrition Journal* 2004;3:9. doi:10.1186/1475–2891-3-9.

You're fat because you eat too much.

False again. The truth is, we aren't fat because we eat too much; we eat too much because we're fat. Being fat means that fat is trapped in the fat cells by high insulin levels and cannot escape to be metabolized for energy. An obese person is literally starving at the cellular level because he or she can't burn his or her own fat for fuel. And the obese person (or even slightly overweight person) didn't get fat by simply eating too much. He or she got fat by eating the wrong things. What things? Foods that increase glucose and insulin production, like "healthy grains."

Fructose is good for you.

Everyone loves fructose. What's not to love? It's natural and it's delicious. Many parents steer their children away from unhealthy sucrose-laden sodas and encourage them to drink healthier fruit juices instead. Many children's drinks use the presence of "real fruit juice" as a selling point, suggesting that a drink made primarily from fruit juice is fundamentally healthy.

Fructose and things containing fructose frequently appear on lists of low glycemic foods because fructose doesn't cause the increase in blood glucose that most other carbohydrates do.

The net result of all this is that well-intentioned parents and others (like schools and day care centers) give fruit juice, lots of fruit juice, to children, thinking it's a good thing. I've even seen diabetic cookbooks that advocate using fructose instead of sucrose in baking.

Lots of fruit juice *is* a good thing, *if* your plan is to help you or your child get a head start on heart disease[1] and diabetes.[2]

What's different about fructose?

Unlike most other sugars that are metabolized through a glucose response in the bloodstream, fructose is metabolized directly in the liver. Fructose consumption at today's typical levels causes the liver to produce excess triglycerides. Not just a few extra triglycer-

---

1. Seneff, S, et al., Is the metabolic syndrome caused by a high fructose, and relatively low fat, low cholesterol diet? *Archives of Medical Science* 2011; 7, 1: 8–20.

2. Johnson, R, et al., Could Excessive Fructose Intake and Uric Acid Cause Type 2 Diabetes? *Endocrinology Review* 2009; 30(1): 96–116.

ides—a bunch of them,[1] which is ill-advised for anyone, including children. Fructose also causes the cells in the body to become increasingly resistant to insulin, hastening onset of Type 2 diabetes (or worsening it in those who are already insulin-resistant).[2]

It's ironic that those who have recently become very vocal against high fructose corn syrup will think nothing of drinking a huge, fructose-laden glass of fruit juice. In doing so, they are overlooking the fact that it's nothing more than the added fructose that turns *corn syrup* into the often indicted *high fructose corn syrup*.

How should we deal with fructose? I say avoid it as much as possible. For me, this means

- Avoiding fruit juices of any kind.
- Avoiding anything containing high fructose corn syrup (this is pretty easy to do if you avoid processed foods entirely, which is always advisable).
- Eat fresh fruit in great moderation—an apple here or there isn't a problem for most people, but eating tons of fruit day in and day out or loading the blender for low-fat fruit smoothies every day is too much fructose for anyone.

Grains are an important part of a healthy diet.

I've saved this one for last because there has probably been no greater lie in the history of health and nutrition than the propagation of the "healthy grains" message. The contention that human beings need to eat grains is hogwash.

I'll be as unabashed as I can be: Grains, most notably wheat, have no place in the human diet.

When I say that aloud, I typically hear the response, "but there are a million studies out there showing that grains are healthy."

---

1. Especially in men: Couchepin, C, et al., Markedly Blunted Metabolic Effects of Fructose in Healthy Young Female Subjects Compared With Male Subjects. *Diabetes Care* 2008; 31:1254–1256.

2. Basciano, H, et al., Fructose, insulin resistance, and metabolic dyslipidemia. *Nutrition & Metabolism* 2005 Feb 21;2(1):5.

It's true that many studies show improved health with higher intake of whole grains on issues from heart disease to blood pressure to birth defects. But healthier in relation to whom? Healthier than people who get an equivalent amount of fiber and nutrients from vegetables? No.

Instead of comparing a group of people who eat grains to those who have replaced grains with vegetables, nuts, and berries, these studies compare people who eat highly refined grains or sugar-laden junk foods to those who eat whole grains. Of course, whole grains are healthier than highly refined grains.

So I suggest you ask "In relation to what?" when you hear claims about something being "healthful" or "good for you."

The real question is this: How healthy are whole grains compared to no grains? Stated another way, are whole grains intrinsically healthful or harmful?

As I was writing this book I came across *Wheat Belly* by William Davis, which documents the harmful effects of wheat in our diet.

The fundamental premise of *Wheat Belly* is that the wheat we eat today is very different genetically from the wheat of 50 years ago, due to cross-breeding and genetic manipulation. The result are strains of wheat that are not only unproven as safe, but are shown in a wide array of studies to be quite harmful, not just to those people with diagnosed celiac disease, but to everyone.

Here are some of the important points Dr. Davis makes:

- 75% of the supposedly healthy complex carbohydrates in wheat is the chain of glucose molecules known as amylopectin A, which is more readily digested than any other carbohydrate forms. This causes wheat (even whole-grain wheat) to induce glucose spikes in the bloodstream that are greater than those from any other carbohydrate, including sucrose.

- Glutens (wheat proteins) are so similar to naturally occurring proteins in the human body that they play havoc with the immune system, and not just in those people diagnosed with celiac disease.

- Lectins (sugar-binding proteins) in the wheat are believed to be the cause of intestinal leakage (i.e., "leaky gut"), whereby proteins enter the bloodstream and cause an unfavorable immune response, leading to inflammation and autoimmune disorders, as discussed in Chapter 4.
- In addition to the proteins in the wheat gluten, there are more than 1,000 other proteins in wheat, many of which show alarming association with a variety of disorders, including autoimmune disease, liver disease, and neurological impairment.
- The clearest link between wheat and illness is shown in people with immune-mediated gluten intolerance, known more commonly as celiac disease. According to Dr. Davis, however, only 10% of people with celiac disease are diagnosed, leaving the other 90% unaware of the dangers caused by the wheat proteins that they are eating.
- Traditional tests for celiac disease check for an immune response to only a few wheat proteins, ignoring the 1,000 or so proteins in wheat that are capable of causing the same damaging effects as the few that are tested for.
- What might be most alarming, however, is that a person does not have to have traditional symptoms of celiac disease in order to experience the harmful effects of the wheat proteins. These "latent" sufferers lack the traditional, acute symptoms of celiac disease (i.e., cramping, diarrhea, severe nutrient malabsorption) yet experience a harmful immune system reaction to wheat proteins.
- "Gluten-mediated reactions have been documented to affect every organ in the human body, sparing none. Eyes, brain, sinuses, lungs, bones... you name it, gluten antibodies have been there"—Dr. Davis.

For those of you over 40, think back 25 years—do you remember there being the huge number of wheat-sensitive people back then that there are today? Do you remember "wheat-free" zones or warnings on packages that the product contains wheat? According to *Wheat Belly*, the percentage of people with celiac disease has doubled in the past 20 years and increased fourfold in the past 50 years; in fact, tests on blood samples saved from decades past prove that it's not due to improvements in our ability to detect the disease.

I urge you to read *Wheat Belly*—especially if you are skeptical about the contention that wheat is harmful.

I found more interesting information in an article in the British Journal of Nutrition on the inflammatory nature of lectins from grains, via molecular mimicry (ingested foods appearing to the immune system as bodily structures), specifically as they contribute to rheumatoid arthritis.

The authors, Cordain et al. noted, and I'm translating here, say that when you eat grains, your intestines get leaky and the proteins from the grains leak through into your bloodstream, where they are recognized as foreign invaders by the immune system. Moreover, in most people over age 40, the increasingly fatigued immune system not only attacks the proteins from the grains but it also attacks the structurally similar proteins that play a significant role in synovial function, resulting in rheumatoid arthritis.[1] Whenever I encounter anyone who suffers from rheumatoid arthritis, I can't help but wonder how much of their pain could be alleviated if they stopped eating grains, especially wheat.

This mechanism is repeated in different scenarios in which proteins in certain foods, traveling through a leaky gut, cause an immune response against healthy, non-threatening body tissues.

In my research, I've learned that "healthy whole grains" are implicated in nearly every facet of our current health woes, from diabetes to heart disease to mental illness. I applaud Dr. Davis for his insights and his dedication to exposing wheat's harmful effects. I hope he sells 50 million copies.

If you are interested in being healthier, I urge you try giving up all grains for 90 days and see how you feel.[2] I suspect that you'll be very surprised at the array of ailments that improve. What do you

---

1. Cordain, et al. Modulation of immune function by dietary lectins in rheumatoid arthritis. *British Journal of Nutrition* 2000;83, 207–217.

2. But like Dr. Davis cautions, don't give up eating whole grains by substituting "gluten-free foods," because they're typically loaded with extremely high glycemic starches that will send your glucose levels into the stratosphere.

have to lose? Certainly not vital nutrients, especially if you replace the grains with vegetables, nuts, and berries.

THE MOST IMPORTANT POINTS FROM THIS CHAPTER

- Your grandmother was right: Veggies are good for you.
- Processed, nitrite-laden meats have no place in a healthy diet.
- The best thing to do with processed foods is avoid them altogether.
- Fruits are best in great moderation and avoid fruit juices and fructose-sweetened products altogether.
- Saturated fats are not the demon that mainstream thinking paints them to be. The biggest dangers with saturated fats is not the fats themselves; it's what we do to them: oxidize them with over-cooking and eat them in the presence of excessively high blood glucose levels, both of which produce damaging advanced glycated end products.
- There is no place for grains in the human diet. Wheat, the most damaging of all, should be entirely avoided in any form. I have yet to find a single study that shows a diet containing grains is healthier than an otherwise equivalent diet that replaces grains with vegetables, nuts, and berries.
- Avoid pesticide-laden and genetically modified foods.

7

Setting Goals

This is where the rubber meets the road, as they say. Everything before this chapter has been background information designed to make it clear why these changes are necessary. This chapter will help you turn these generic concepts into specific goals. The next chapter will help you devise a plan of action to meet your goals.

Verify the Results

You can read all the research studies, how-to books, motivational websites, and magazine articles about health that you want. You can even talk to every physician on the planet, but the only way to absolutely know whether what you are doing is improving your health is to verify the results through testing.

For example, some studies say that saturated fat is bad for anyone, some say that it's good for everyone, and some say that there is so much variability in the way we, as individuals, metabolize saturated fats that discussions about whether saturated fats are healthy are meaningless. While my research on the subject shows considerable flaws in the "saturated fat is bad" dogma that has permeated dietary advice for decades, there's no doubt in my mind that a small percentage of people metabolize saturated fats less effectively than others and for these people, eating too much saturated fat at one time can lead to unfavorable lipid production for the hours following that meal. This is especially relevant to those who already have heart disease.

Because of this individual variability, the only way to know for sure what is ideal is to eat a controlled diet for a month or two and have a lipid VAP, NMR, or other lipid subfraction test and see what your lipids have done. If your lipid subfractions are favorable, then you know that you've been eating favorably for you. If your lipid analysis was unfavorable, you can try adjusting your diet, perhaps with more fat, perhaps eating less fat, and test again. How did your lipid tests change? Did they get better or worse? Anyone's opinion about how you should eat could be wrong, but numbers from a lab rarely lie.

Another powerful indicator is to measure how your triglyceride levels respond to a specific meal. While this is a task that requires somewhat more effort, it can certainly be worth it, as I describe in *Achieving Triglyceride Goals* on page 136.

Establishing a Baseline

If you don't know where you started, you won't know how far you've come. By this I mean for everything you want to improve, it's exceedingly useful to measure before you start making changes. It sounds obvious, but it's something that's easily overlooked. Few of us would forget to record our weight and body fat percentage before we started a new diet, but when you start talking about improving your Omega-3 Index or measuring your lipid particle counts, or any one of the dozens of other things I've advocated monitoring, a baseline (a starting value, before making any changes) is even more important.

I recognize that not all of you are in a position to finish this book and dash out to LabCorp for a battery of baseline tests. Recognize, however, that the more you can document before beginning, the better you will be at measuring improvement. At a bare minimum, I would suggest that in addition to obtaining your physician's endorsement for any lifestyle and exercise changes, you obtain the following baseline data:

- Body weight and body fat percentage[1]
- Coronary calcium scan
- Fasting glucose
- Fasting insulin
- A1C
- Lipid subfraction analysis (e.g., LipoScience or VAP)
- High-resolution or "cardiac" C-reactive protein (hsCRP)
- Omega-3 Index
- A quantity of 10 or more blood pressure readings taken at different times over a period of days (one reading is not enough to get a valid picture of your blood pressure)[2]
- Vitamin D, 25-Hydroxy vitamin D level (see Appendix B)
- Comprehensive metabolic panel (CMP)

---

1. I advocate recording your starting body weight and body fat percentage *not* because these should be something that you target specifically but rather, they should be something that you enjoy watching improve.

2. Consult a reliable testing source to ensure that you buy a good electronic blood pressure meter. Or, better yet, if your ears and eyes are good enough, buy a blood pressure cuff and a stethoscope and learn how to take blood pressure without electronics.

If your physician wasn't involved in obtaining these tests, be sure and share the results so that the two of you can use them as a foundation for your plan of action.

Recapping the Major Foes

As you may recall from page 107, I have focused my personal preventive health strategy on the following areas:

- Controlling blood glucose levels
- Preventing inflammation from occurring
- Reducing existing inflammation
- Optimizing lipid health (i.e., increasing LDL particle size, reducing LDL particle count, increasing HDL, and reducing triglycerides)

I try to implement changes that benefit as many of these categories as possible. Fortunately, it's common for things that help one area to also benefit others. For example, optimizing our omega-6 to omega-3 intake will not only reduce inflammation but will also improve our lipids (by lowering triglycerides) and help our glucose metabolism by producing healthier cell membranes that enable the glucose receptors to more effectively transport glucose into and out of the cells.

Goals of a Healthy Lifestyle

I'm not comfortable with vague, feel-good measures that make me think I'm living healthy lifestyles without quantifiable proof. To me, pursuing optimum health is about defining specific, measurable goals and working to achieve them.

Based upon what I've learned, I've broken the general concept of *preventive health* into a specific list of goals[1] that I can measure myself against. My personal goals are very aggressive. How aggressive you choose to set your goals is up to your situation and your personality.

Just Because They're My Goals Doesn't Mean They Must Be Yours

Common sense alert: Just because I've included my personal goals in this chapter doesn't mean they should automatically be your goals. Everyone is different and what's reasonable for me to achieve may not be reasonable for you to achieve.

This is where an effective partnership with a like-minded physician is valuable so that the two of you can chart a course optimized for your needs. For example, if you have very little family history of heart disease and your coronary calcium scan (see *The Coronary Calcium Scan* on page 18) shows no evidence of coronary plaque, you may decide that your lipid goals do not need to be as strict as mine. Similarly, if you are already significantly insulin-resistant, my fasting and postprandial glucose goals might simply be unattainable for you (or if you're young and have no insulin resistance, you can probably achieve my glucose goals quite easily). What's important is that you set meaningful goals for yourself and consistently measure your progress against them.

Unfortunately, many physicians don't value such things as effective glucose control, lipid subfraction analysis, and omega-6 and omega-3 levels. If you care about this, it's up to you to find a physician who does too. Believe me, they're out there. You just have to find one. See *Find a Partner* on page 173 for some thoughts on finding a prevention-minded physician.

Like any goal, some of these goals are more elusive than others. Fortunately, they can start paying dividends in better health as soon as your values begin improving, long before they reach an optimum range.

---

1. Many of my goals are influenced by the work of Dr. Davis, author of *The Heart Scan Blog*, *Track Your Plaque*, and *Wheat Belly* and the founder of the *Track Your Plaque* web community. Dr. Davis is a pioneer in the field of preventive cardiac care. You owe it to yourself to study his work.

As you pursue these improvements, remember also that some will take longer than others. For example, I saw my triglycerides drop more than 90% in about a month, but it took a couple of months to start seeing measurable improvements in my fasting glucose. Be patient and give your body time to heal. Testing is vital but testing too often can be frustrating and expensive. I'll provide some guidelines for how often to test certain things but much of that depends on how unhealthy your lab values are, how aggressively you're making changes, your ability to afford the testing, among other factors.

Let's look at some specific goals and how you might go about reaching them.

Lipid Health

You may think it's odd that after spending so much time disputing the lipid hypothesis, I would have specific goals for lipid health. If you read the lipid chapter and the Appendix A carefully, though, you'll see that I believe that my lipid health is central to my cardiac health. It's just that the lipid hypothesis that blames total cholesterol, or even just LDL and HDL levels, on heart disease, is oversimplified and needs to be replaced with a model that accounts for lipid subfractions.

Note that some of my lipid goals include measurements specific to LipoScience's NMR technology, namely the LDL particle count and LDL small particle count. If you elect to base your goals upon another subfraction analysis (e.g., Berkeley HeartLab or Atherotech's VAP), the clinical guideline literature available from their websites (see *Where to Learn More* on page 253) would be an effective starting place for defining goals that are specific to each company's subfraction technology.

Optimizing our lipids is perhaps the trickiest goal of all, due to the incredible variability between people. One thing I will never say to anyone is "if you do x, then y will absolutely happen." I will, however, tell you what I've discovered and what I've learned by monitoring how these changes have affected my lipid health.

This is very much a situation that requires us to study the many variables, investigate and try different options, and most of all measure the results of our actions with lipid subfraction analysis and other means so that we can make the appropriate course corrections.

As with many of the recommended lifestyle changes here, some lipid-optimizing efforts will likely have multiple benefits. For example, the vitamin B3 (niacin) can increase HDL and decrease LDL, all while lowering particle count and small particle count.[1] Similarly, omega-3 fish oil can reduce triglycerides and improve LDL and HDL.[2]

Note: It's likely that you've never actually had your LDL measured, despite what you and your doctor think. First as a result of technical limitations and now to save your insurance company money, traditional cholesterol tests estimate the amount of LDL in your blood using HDL and triglyceride levels—they don't actually measure LDL. Depending on your level of HDL and triglycerides, the LDL value you receive from a traditional cholesterol test can be quite inaccurate. See Appendix H for important information on how to properly measure your true LDL level.

---

1. Niacin, in its many available forms, can be confusing and its skin flushing side effects can be alarming. See Appendix G more information.

2. LOVAZA (omega-3-acid ethyl esters) prescribing information; GlaxoSmithKline; Research Triangle Park, NC 27709. See Appendix M for information on obtaining omega-3 fish oil via prescription versus over the counter.

Triglyceride Goals

Attribute	Goal	Notes
Triglycerides, fasting	< 60 mg/dL	This is an aggressive goal. Many people are satisfied with fasting triglycerides below 100 mg/dL. It all depends on how aggressive you want to be. That decision will likely be a product of how much cardiac plaque your calcium scan reveals.
Triglycerides, postprandial	< 100 mg/dL	Triglyceride levels typically peak between three and four hours after eating. This is an aggressive goal. Someone with no coronary plaque may be comfortable letting postprandial triglycerides reach higher levels.

Triglycerides are a key factor in optimizing cardiac health. If your body is producing an unfavorable amount of triglycerides, it's far more likely that you will develop arterial plaque.

In cases of excessively high triglycerides, the liver can develop non-alcoholic fatty liver disease,[1] which will cause the liver to be dysfunctional, further contributing to unfavorable lipid production. And if triglycerides get too high, they can even damage the pancreas, which contributes to poor glucose metabolism, which brings a host of related complications.

Achieving Triglyceride Goals

For most people, the primary causes of elevated triglycerides are grains (especially wheat) and sugar (especially fructose). Many people also report that eliminating vegetable oils lower their triglycerides. As with blood glucose levels, optimizing your triglyceride levels requires that you stop eating the foods that ele-

1. The incidence of nonalcoholic fatty liver disease has increased dramatically in the United States, doubling from about 5.5% to 11% between 1988 and 2008. How do you fatten a person's liver? The same way you fatten a goose's liver so that you can make tasty goose liver pate: feed it lots and lots of grains.

vate triglycerides and begin eating foods (and consider taking supplements) that help your body achieve healthy triglyceride levels.

I keep drawing parallels between blood glucose levels and lipid health because you'll likely find, as I did, that the same dietary modifications that improve glucose levels also improve lipid health. That is, "eating to your meter" (eating to minimize blood glucose levels) will prevent unfavorable glucose spikes and will likely also improve your triglycerides.

For nearly everyone, eliminating grains, sugars, and vegetable oils while maintaining an effective blood glucose level will considerably improve triglyceride levels. Adding some omega-3 fish oil will also help you lower your triglyceride levels, too.

If you've read Chapter 3 on diabetes, you know that there are very different implications for our fasting glucose versus our postprandial glucose. Watching only fasting glucose and ignoring what our glucose does after eating is missing a very big part of the picture.

Similarly, watching only our fasting triglycerides ignores a very important part of lipid health: what are our triglyceride levels doing after eating a typical meal? This is an important question, especially for those battling heart disease, because dietary fats are made primarily from triglycerides and how quickly and effectively we break down these triglyceride-laden particles plays a role in the formation of coronary plaque. Consuming more than our body can effectively metabolize will result in the formation of small, unfavorable lipid particles instead of larger beneficial particles. For most people, this isn't an issue, as the majority of us can easily handle the dietary fats in most any meal. A problem arises, however, for those having a compromised liver (perhaps from insulin resistance that has diminished the liver's ability to effectively metabolize dietary fats). For such people, it's important to know what the safe threshold is for a given meal.

I spent months pleased with my impressively low fasting triglycerides while struggling to understand why my LDL particle counts weren't as low as I expected. The key to better LDL particle counts for me turned out to be controlling my postprandial triglyceride levels. Learning how to do that meant studying how my triglycerides responded to specific types of foods in the three to five hours after eating.[1]

Because triglyceride levels typically peak 3 to 4 hours after eating and return to normal a couple of hours after that, virtually everyone is in a non-fasting state from breakfast time until five or six hours after their last bite of food at night (which for most people is a few hours after dinner). The result is that very few people spend more than 4 or 5 hours a day in the fasting state, and for most people the number is far less.

I contend that what is happening 19 or 20 hours a day influences our health way more than what's happening the other 4 or 5 hours a day. As with blood glucose, it's very possible to have fasting triglyceride levels that are favorable but have routinely elevated postprandial triglyceride levels. Levels that are high enough to significantly contribute to cardiac plaque formation.

Unfortunately, measuring postprandial triglycerides is more complicated and expensive than measuring postprandial glucose levels. This is because:

- It's impossible to predict exactly when triglycerides will peak after a meal, though they typically do so three to four hours after eating.
- A standard lipid panel, even if purchased on sale from one of the online vendors listed in Appendix S, can cost $20 to $45.

This means if you want to use traditional laboratory testing to check your postprandial triglyceride levels for a given meal, you would have to purchase three or four lipid panels and have your

1. Dr. Davis has written an insightful paper on the subject of postprandial lipid response. "The Lipid Challenge" provides information on the usefulness of measuring postprandial triglyceride levels, including suggestions for performing specific tests with known quantities of various types of fats. This paper alone is sufficient justification for joining his *Track Your Plaque* online cardiac health forum. This sort of thinking illustrates perfectly how superior self-testing is compared to all of the speculation and research out there.

local LabCorp draw your blood three or four times, 15 to 20 minutes apart, beginning three hours after your meal. This would be inconvenient and prohibitively expensive (at least to me). Not to mention that the local LabCorp is probably accustomed to people having fasting lipid testing, and if you tried to explain that you were measuring postprandial triglyceride levels in order to determine how effectively your body converts unfavorable triglycerides into more favorable lipid particles, they'd probably look at you like you had lobsters growing out of your ears.

A more reasonable approach is purchasing a CardioChek meter and some triglyceride test strips. This handy meter is about the size of a paperback book and can check your triglycerides (or HDL or LDL, depending on which test strips you purchase) in the comfort of your home, with a simple finger stick. The test strips for triglycerides are about $4.00 each, which is much more cost-effective than purchasing four or five LabCorp lipid panels to try and catch a peak triglyceride level.

Using LabCorp as a comparison, I checked the accuracy of the CardioChek meter and found it to be acceptable. It was off only by 2 or 3 mg/dL on two out of three comparisons and was off by about 10 mg/dL on the third comparison. While not perfect, this is probably good enough for determining if a meal is sending your triglycerides to 100 mg/dL or if it's sending them all the way to 200 or 300 mg/dL.

Much as with self-glucose testing, a postprandial triglyceride check is vital to optimizing what you eat, most likely along the lines of what types of fats and what quantity is ideal for you, based upon your postprandial triglyceride goal. This effort showed me that I'm someone who doesn't metabolize saturated fats as effectively as most people. For example, by choosing a maximum postprandial triglyceride level of 100 mg/dL, I use this specific, objective threshold to determine what saturated fat intake will keep me within that limit. By testing myself as I've described, I know that I have no problem enjoying a thick, juicy steak from a grass-fed cow but I probably don't want to follow the meal with a glass of eggnog made from 12 ounces of heavy whipping cream and six raw eggs.

In summary, the best approach to reducing one's triglycerides is

- Eliminate grains, replacing them with vegetables, nuts, and berries.
- Minimize carbohydrates (especially fructose), eating them in sufficient moderation so as to never cause unfavorable glucose levels.
- Consider supplementing your diet with omega-3 fatty acids from fish oil.[1]
- Speak to your physician about supplementing with niacin to help optimize your triglycerides.[2]
- All of the above steps will very effectively control your fasting triglycerides. To really take it to the next level, buy a CardioChek triglyceride meter to measure your body's response to different types of meals to identify exactly how sensitive your body is to specific types and quantities of fats. If you perform a small series of these carefully controlled tests, you'll have infinitely more clarity on how to optimize your diet for the best possible postprandial triglyceride production (this will be especially valuable in determining whether saturated fat is good for you and at what level).

  If you take this extra step to study your postprandial triglyceride level, you'll have significant insight into your optimum diet, far more than attempting to adjust your diet based upon a population study or even a clinical study.

LDL Goals

Because I have the most experience with LipoScience's NMR lipid subfraction analysis, my LDL goals are stated in terms of the particle count and small particle count categories defined by LipoScience and unique to their testing methods. Recall that there are a variety of technologies for analyzing lipid subfractions (e.g.,

---

1. See Appendix M for some more information on supplementing with omega-3 fatty acids and how over-the-counter fish oils compare to prescription omega-3 fish oil product, Lovasa.

2. Niacin is wonderful stuff. It improves HDL, LDL, and triglycerides. See Appendix G for information on supplementing with niacin.

Berkeley HeartLab, Atherotech's VAP), each with their own subfraction categories and clinical guidelines.

Attribute	Goal	Notes
LDL-P (LDL Particle Count)	< 800 nmol/L	An analogous, though not identical, measurement in the VAP test would be $apoB_{100}$.
LDL Small Particle Count	< 200 nmol/L	To obtain an analogous, though not identical, measurement in the VAP test, add the values for LDL_4 and LDL_3.
LDL Particle Size	> 20.5 nm	Size does matter! Larger LDL particles are better for you than small ones.
LDL-C (Total LDL Cholesterol)	55–60 mg/dL	Unlike HDL, which I try to get as high as possible, I *do not* want my LDL as low as possible. I just aim for an LDL-C that is less than 60 mg/dL. This is because *excessively* low LDL-C levels are associated with increased cancer rates, dementia, and other undesirable conditions.

As discussed extensively in Chapter 2, the total amount of LDL (also known as LDL-C), is far less relevant to cardiac risk than LDL particles (primarily small LDL particles, according to some leading-edge cardiologists). The goal of an effective lifestyle is to *minimize* LDL particle count, *maximize* LDL size, and *optimize* total LDL (LDL-C). This doesn't mean that simply driving LDL-C down as low as possible is the solution—keep the total LDL picture in mind when assessing lipid health.

A little common sense is warranted here. I'm not saying that the total amount of LDL is *completely* irrelevant. After all, if someone's LDL is 300 mg/dL, it's very unlikely that this person is going to have a favorable particle count. It's just not possible that a total LDL value that high would be able to be stored in a healthy number of LDL particles.

What's wrong with the current approach, however, is that too many people are focusing solely on total LDL, trying simply to drive that number lower and lower, with complete disregard for LDL particle count. This can cause LDL levels that appear healthy but are actually unfavorable, due to high particle count, or can cause LDL values that appear to be unhealthy to actually be favorable or benign, due to a low particle count.

Achieving LDL Goals

At the risk of sounding like a broken record, the very same things that minimize glucose and triglyceride levels will also help optimize LDL. The biggest culprit in producing unfavorable LDL particles is wheat, hands down. All grains, but most notably wheat, will cause your LDL characteristics to shift from larger, fewer particles to smaller, more numerous particles.

What about the studies that show that whole grains improve LDL? Every such study I've read compares a diet containing whole grains to a diet containing refined grains and sugars. I've never seen a study that compares LDL levels between people who eat whole grains and people who have entirely replaced grains in their diets with vegetables, nuts, and berries. I'm confident that such a study would show that whole grains are inferior to a healthy diet devoid of grains. My personal experience certainly bears this out. Not to mention that the "grains help LDL" studies that I've seen are looking at LDL-C (total LDL), not LDL particle count, which is a far more relevant indicator of LDL health.

The approach I take for optimizing LDL is the following:

- Eliminate grains, replacing them with vegetables, nuts, and berries.
- Minimize unfavorable carbohydrates (especially sugar, including fructose).
- Speak to your physician about supplementing with niacin to help optimize your LDL. Niacin has proven vital in helping me achieve my LDL goals, specifically in reducing my LDL particle count and LDL small particle count.

HDL Goals

Attribute	Goal	Notes
HDL-C (Total HDL Cholesterol)	> 60 mg/dL	I try and achieve an HDL-C that is as high as possible.
HDL-P	> 34.9 umol/L	Inversely to LDL-P (particle count), which we want to be low, we want the HDL-P to be high. Studies have shown that HDL-P is a better indicator than HDL-C in predicting the risk of coronary artery disease.
HDL Size	> 9.6 nm	Like LDL, larger particles are better than smaller ones.

In the grand scale of the lipid battlefield, HDL is generally regarded as the good guy. Beyond that, however, researchers are learning more and more about optimizing HDL far beyond the simple "more is better" philosophy.

If you do want to keep things simple, you can set your HDL goal as any HDL-C value above your desired range and leave it at that. (My HDL goal is rather aggressive. Many sources consider anything above 45 mg/dL a healthy HDL level.) If, on the other hand, you want to optimize your HDL even further, you can start looking at the size of the HDL (larger is better) and the HDL particle count (more is better). Some studies have shown that, like LDL, the HDL particle count is a more reliable indicator of HDL health than simply looking at total HDL (HDL-C).

Achieving HDL Goals

Improving HDL is a bit trickier than improving triglycerides and LDL. For whatever reason, HDL seems to change more slowly in response to dietary and lifestyle changes. Because of this, it's tougher to identify cause and effect when it comes to HDL; the lag between diet or lifestyle changes and the HDL response is frequently too great to make it clear what improved HDL and what did not.

That said, I've come to believe that the following will help most people's HDL

- Exercise[1]
- All the changes that help triglycerides and LDL
- Avoiding low-fat diets

General Suggestions for Optimizing Lipid Health

The common thread permeating these sections on optimizing triglycerides, LDL, and HDL is to remove grains from the diet. The three biggest culprits in the formation of unhealthy lipids are grains, vegetable oils, and sugar (especially fructose).

My suggestion to anyone interested in optimizing lipid health is to:

- Eliminate grains, replacing them with vegetables, nuts, and berries.
- Avoid all vegetable oils.
- Include plenty of fat in your diet, moderating saturated fats only in the unlikely event that postprandial triglyceride analysis indicates that you produce unfavorable levels of triglycerides in response to a significant intake of saturated fat.
- Carefully control your blood glucose levels to avoid damaging glucose spikes.
- Optimize your intake of omega-3 fatty acids and minimize your intake of omega-6 fatty acids.
- Exercise to benefit your HDL.
- Avoid fructose, except for the small amount in berries and the occasional fruit.

---

1. Exactly how much exercise and exactly what type best optimizes HDL is not perfectly clear, but the general consensus is that exercise doesn't have to be extremely intense to benefit HDL and other lipids. For example, moderate exercise (e.g., jogging at a pace of 10–11 minutes per mile for 20 minutes at a time) has been shown to benefit HDL just as much as exercising far more vigorously.

- Use lipid subfraction analysis to monitor your lipid health, adjusting your diet as necessary to find what works best for you.
- Partner with a physician who shares your enthusiasm for optimizing your lipids in this way.

Glucose and Insulin

Numerous studies have shown that even moderately elevated glucose levels are damaging to a variety of systems in the body. These damaging effects are so insidious and so preventable that I include blood sugar control in every discussion on preventive health.

Remember, every single moment that your glucose level exceeds the optimal range, your body is being damaged.

Glucose and Insulin Goals

Attribute	Goal	Notes
Blood Glucose, fasting	< 85 mg/dL	This is an aggressive fasting glucose that may be unreachable by many adults today.
Blood Glucose, postprandial	< 100 mg/dL	My goal is to never allow my blood glucose level to exceed 100 mg/dL. This includes my glucose levels one and two hours after eating, which are typically the highest levels one sees. Someone with excessive insulin resistance may simply not be able to achieve postprandial levels this low.
A1C	< 5.0%	Even with its inherent flaws, I still aim for an A1C value below 5%.
Insulin, fasting	2–6 uIU/mL	The lower the fasting insulin level is, the less insulin-resistant you likely are.

For those who are so severely insulin-resistant that their blood glucose is in an unhealthy range even when fasting (e.g., fasting glucose levels over 110 or 120 mg/dL), controlling glucose levels becomes far more difficult, as practically any food at all will increase blood glucose to a damaging level. In such cases, and in cases of Type 1 diabetics who make no insulin whatsoever, extremely rigid blood sugar control is even more vital. *Dr. Bernstein's Diabetes Solution* contains valuable advice on how anyone, insulin-dependent or not, can rigidly yet safely control blood sugar.

Depending on how insulin-resistant you are, your blood glucose goals may need to be higher if you cannot reach a postprandial level as low as you would like. If this is the case, don't be discouraged. Any reduction toward the optimal goal will help you reduce your insulin resistance, which will, in time, help you reach still more favorable postprandial glucose levels.

Insulin resistance, which goes hand in hand with increased blood sugars, is the other edge of the double-edged sword that is Type 2 diabetes. As insulin resistance increases, increasing average insulin levels cause damage of their own, distinct from the damage caused by elevated glucose levels.

The terms *insulin resistance* and *insulin sensitivity* refer to the same thing.

As we approach Type 2 diabetes, we become more resistant to insulin's effects, thereby making us less sensitive to insulin.

Some supplements are reported to be effective in helping some people increase insulin sensitivity. One of these is r-lipoic acid, an over-the-counter supplement in the United States that is a prescription medication in Europe. R-lipoic acid is an "insulin mimetic," meaning it tricks the body into thinking that there's more insulin in the bloodstream than there really is, causing the body to produce a bit less insulin. This can help reduce insulin resistance in some, but not all, people. You may see this product listed as "alpha-lipoic acid," which is a 50/50 mixture of r-lipoic acid and l-lipoic acid. Studies show that the r-lipoic acid is much better absorbed, so I purchase the pure r-lipoic acid rather than the alpha-lipoic acid mixture. If you are insulin-resistant, consider discussing the potential benefits of r-lipoic acid with your physician.

Note that if you are extremely insulin-resistant, you may be very far from this ideal range and achieving it may not be possible. In such a case, focus less on the overall fasting insulin level and instead use the amount of reduction over time as an indication of your progress toward improved health. For example, if your fasting insulin level drops from 25 uUI/mL to 15 uUI/mL over six months or a year, you know that you're making progress. Even though you haven't reached an "ideal" range, you'll still benefit from such a dramatic improvement.

Achieving Glucose and Insulin Goals

The single best way to control blood glucose levels is to stop eating foods that elevate your blood glucose.

It sounds simple, and it is. The biggest problem with controlling blood glucose through diet is this: *Doing so requires that you ignore the advice of experts who tell you to get 60% or more of your calories from grains.* In fact, their advice is exactly what's been causing our blood glucose to go up every time we eat, causing us to gain weight and form cardiac plaque.

If you want to ensure that you're eating in a healthy way, you must purchase and use a blood glucose meter regularly. If you follow any diet, be it mine, The Zone, Atkins, Weight Watchers, South Beach, or you just "eat well most of the time," and you don't monitor your blood sugar one hour and two hours after a meal, *you cannot be sure that your eating habits are preventing damaging glucose spikes.*

In *Blood Sugar 101,* Jenny Ruhl calls this "eating to your meter" and that's exactly what it is: letting your one- and two-hour finger stick glucose readings be your guide to the suitability of the foods you're eating.

Oh, no! This sounds obsessive. This sounds like I'm treating myself like a diabetic. I'm not a diabetic!

Yes, I had some of the same reactions when I realized what effective glucose control requires. But it's not as onerous as it sounds. You probably don't eat the variety of foods that you think you do. Most people have "favorite" foods that they return to time and again, with the net result that 80% of what they eat is probably represented by ten or twenty different food items. It doesn't take long to determine how your favorite foods affect your blood glucose and either move them to an *acceptable* list or an *unacceptable* list as you modify your eating habits.

Just a couple of weeks with your glucose meter and you'll have a very good idea of which foods are your friends and which are not. For example, a few strawberries might not send your blood glucose over 110 mg/dL but a large glass of milk may.

It doesn't take long to relearn how to "eat to your meter" and keep your blood glucose below your established goal. Trust me—your body will thank you for it. And whatever you do, please don't believe that you can blindly use a glycemic index chart to determine what's going to be safe for your blood glucose levels. The problems with glycemic index charts are too numerous to detail, but they include the following:

- We are all different in how we respond to certain foods. Foods that don't cause my blood glucose to go above 100 mg/dL could send yours to 175.
- Differences in food preparation can dramatically affect how much of a glycemic response a food causes.
- Fruits and vegetables can have different glycemic indices depending on season, crop, cultivation methods, and other factors.
- Fructose, typically touted as a healthy sugar by those who don't know any better, is actually quite damaging because it doesn't elevate blood glucose levels or cause an insulin response and therefore typically shows up on lists of low glycemic foods. This allows fructose to sneak in under the radar and cause havoc with the liver.
- People frequently confuse a food's glycemic index with glycemic load. Glycemic index is the tendency, per unit weight or volume, of a food to cause an elevation in blood glucose. Glycemic load is the total amount of impact a typical portion of that food will cause. To illustrate the difference, look at popcorn. Popcorn has a very high glycemic index, but because popcorn isn't very dense, a cup or two of popcorn causes a relatively low glycemic load. (Of course, most people don't eat just a cup or two of popcorn at a time—they eat 10 or 12 cups, typically popped in highly inflammatory omega-6 soybean oil.)

- If a glycemic index table reports that a food is high glycemic, you can probably trust that it's high glycemic. However, don't blindly trust any list that tells you a food is low glycemic until you use your glucose meter to verify its effects on you. Possible exceptions to this are vegetables like spinach and squash and unmodified protein sources like eggs, poultry, seafood, and grass-fed beef. It's still best, however, to use a glucose meter to monitor your response to specific foods until you're sure how your body reacts to each of them.

The good thing about controlling glucose levels is that preventing blood glucose levels from exceeding a healthy level is the single best thing you can do to reduce insulin resistance. The body has a remarkable ability to heal and every single moment you keep your glucose levels in an optimal range, healing is occurring.

As you read in Chapter 3, the vicious cycle of Type 2 diabetes is that the symptom of insulin resistance (elevated blood glucose) causes beta cell death (recall that beta cells are the cells responsible for insulin production) and beta cell death increases the burden on the remaining beta cells, further causing additional beta cells to die.

According to research, pancreatic beta cells can enter a dormant state of impaired function or non-function and stay this way for a while before they die. This provides an opportunity for some beta cell recovery through effective blood glucose controls, which will, in turn, aid in further beta cell recovery. (It's nice to know that the cycles that get us into this mess can also be reversed and help us heal.)

In short, to increase your insulin sensitivity:

- Avoid foods that elevate your blood glucose levels.
- Exercise (weight training is best for this).
- Consider the supplement r-lipoic acid, at a level recommended by your physician. This powerful antioxidant is an insulin mimetic and can help some people reduce insulin resistance.
- Ensure that you are optimizing your omega-3 and omega-6 intake.

Optimize Omega-3 and Omega-6 Levels

As you read in Chapter 4, omega-6 fatty acids are some of the most inflammatory dietary influences. While most of the discussion on omega-6 fats has been in the context of reducing inflammation, another important goal of eating the proper omega-3 to omega-6 ratio is to ensure that the membranes of cells are flexible and pliable, and do not impede the different receptors embedded within them.

Omega-6 and Omega-3 Goals

Attribute	Goal	Notes
Omega-3 Index	> 10%	See page 209 for more information on obtaining this informative, inexpensive test.
Ratio of Omega-6 to Omega-3, in daily intake	1:1, initially; 2:1 after three to six months	As you'll read in this section, it's important to aim not only for an optimal ratio of omega-6 to omega-3 fatty acids, but also to strive to eat the optimal *amount* of each.
Omega-3, daily intake	3 grams of combined DHA and EPA	What I don't get in my food, I supplement with fish oil. Depending on your cardiac history, your omega-3 intake goal may be lower.
Omega-6, daily intake	< 3 grams initially; < 6 grams after three to six months	This intake goal, combined with the omega-3 intake goal, helps ensure the desired 1:1 or 2:1 ratio.

The recognized measure of the omega-3 health is the Omega-3 Index, a test that measures the ratio of omega-3 to omega-6, not within your bloodstream, but within the membranes of your cells, where it's most important. Most Americans have an Omega-3 Index of around 4%. Studies have shown that increasing our Omega-3 Index to above 10 percent results in a 90% reduction in coronary events.[1]

Optimizing Omega-3 and Omega-6 Intake

As you learned in Chapter 4, omega-3 fatty acids are an essential and healthful fatty acid and even though omega-6 fatty acids are also an essential fatty acid, they are required in very small amounts. Indeed, excessive omega-6 intake causes harmful inflammation.

Once again, diet is the key here, but this is a bit trickier because omega-6 fatty acids are *everywhere*. Sadly, they've become a staple in our American diet, thanks primarily to the "experts" who steer us toward things like soybean oil, vegetable oil, safflower oil, and other "heart-healthy" industrial oils. Most people don't realize that there are almost no homogenous sources of fats. What that means is that nearly every source of healthy omega-3 oils also has some omega-6 oil in it, too. This makes controlling our omega-3 and omega-6 intake a bit tricky because it's hard to get one without the other.

To achieve my goal of >10% in the Omega-3 Index, I'm careful to eat so that I'm getting enough omega-3 and not too much omega-6. Doing so requires an effective way of determining how much omega-3 and omega-6 fats are in the foods that I eat. It helps that I avoid processed foods almost entirely, for their packaging typically doesn't reflect omega-6 content. Eating only unprocessed foods (e.g., turkey, chicken, fish, beef, vegetables, nuts) means that it's much easier to monitor my omega-3 and omega-6 intake.

---

1. von Schacky, C, et al. Cardiovascular benefits of omega-3 fatty acids. *Cardiovascular Research* 2007;73:310–315.

For me, achieving an optimal omega-3 and omega-6 balance translates into the following guidelines:

- Each day I ensure that I consume 3 grams of omega-3 fatty acids in the form of EPA and DHA.[1] What I don't obtain in my diet each day, I supplement with omega-3 fish oil. (See Appendix M for more information about obtaining omega-3 fish oil.)

  While in the early stages of restoring my health, I ensured that my daily omega-6 intake didn't exceed my daily omega-3 intake, thus producing a 1:1 omega-6 to omega-3 ratio. This meant limiting my omega-6 intake to no more than three to four grams per day.

- After six months or so, I allowed my omega-6 intake to increase, up to a maximum of 2:1 omega-6 to omega-3 ratio. This means consuming three grams of omega-3 per day and no more than three to six grams of omega-6 fats per day.

  By the way, don't worry about not getting enough omega-6 fatty acids. Omega-6 is so pervasive that it's unavoidable. As a point of comparison, the standard American diet (SAD) typically has an omega-6 to omega-3 ratio of 10:1, 20:1, or even 30:1. The typical American eats 13 grams of omega-6 fatty acids a day![2] I imagine that the makers of anti-inflammatory and blood pressure medications celebrate that!

Just how do you keep track of the total omega-3 and omega-6 intake? There are two approaches you can take:

1. If you want to know exactly how much omega-3 and omega-6 you are consuming daily, I'm afraid there are no shortcuts. You have to know the omega-3 and omega-6 content of everything you eat and track it. There are some great guides out there, in print and on the Internet, which show the omega-3 and omega-6 content of most foods. There also some great software and web-based tools (some of them even free) that contain nutritional information for thousands of food

---

1. The plant-based omega-3 fatty acid, ALA, is so poorly converted by the human body into an effective form that greater than 95% of ALA is wasted. For this reason, I don't count ALA as a bioavailable omega-3 acid. Any ALA I obtain through my diet (i.e., from flax seeds) is just incidental and I don't count it.

2. Tribole, E. *The Ultimate Omega-3 Diet.* New York, NY: McGraw Hill, 2007.

products. (See Appendix L on tools to help if you want to track your food consumption to this level of detail.)

2. You could just take 3 grams of omega-3 fish oil every day and avoid sources of excessive omega-6 fatty acids, based upon reading a list of foods and their omega-3/omega-6 content. Such a book would be the excellent *The Ultimate Omega-3 Diet* by Evelyn Tribole (though I do not agree with the author's unilateral assertion that saturated fat is always bad). This would not be as accurate as tracking everything you eat and calculating the omega-3 to omega-6 ratio, but it's better than 99% of the people out there who gobble omega-6 fatty acids by the tens of grams, and the time you save will allow you to have more of a life than someone like me who spends all his time doing Step 1.

When thinking about omega-3 and omega-6 content, keep in mind that some foods have seemingly horrible ratios of omega-3 to omega-6 but are actually very healthful and some have seemingly good ratios, but are unfavorable. See Appendix T for more information on balancing your omega-3 and omega-6 intake.

Reduce Inflammation

As was made clear in Chapter 4, inflammation plays a central role in overall health, most notably in cardiac health. Blood pressure is a very good indicator of systemic inflammation, as are a variety of inflammatory markers that we can test for in our blood.

Inflammation Goals

Attribute	Goal	Notes
Blood Pressure, resting	< 115, systolic < 70 diastolic	As aggressive as this sounds, even though my starting blood pressures were as high as 145/95 at times, I started seeing blood pressures in the 115/70 range within six months of improved lifestyle.
C-Reactive Protein, as hsCRP (high-sensitivity CRP)	< 1.0 mg/L	CRP is easily affected by such things as not feeling well, insufficient sleep, or a pulled muscle. For this reason, I test periodically but I am more concerned about the general trend rather than any one CRP value.
Homocysteine	< 10 umol/L	See later in this section for information about lowering homocysteine.
Omega-6, daily intake	< 3 grams initially; < 6 grams after three to six months	This intake goal, combined with the omega-3 intake goal, helps ensure the desired 1:1 or 2:1 ratio.
Lp-PLA2	< 200 ng/mL	This inflammatory marker can be lowered with niacin and certain medications.

Regarding homocysteine, some individuals and vitamin suppliers attest to the benefits of B vitamins in lowering homocysteine, but the research I've studied says that lowering homocysteine in this way is just treating the symptom of elevated homocysteine levels and not treating the inflammatory cause of the elevated homocysteine. That is, taking a bunch of B vitamins to lower your homocysteine appears to merely lower homocysteine levels without really reducing inflammation.

One thing to remember: if you're taking niacin (vitamin B3) your homocysteine levels may *increase* as a benign side-effect of the niacin.

Reducing Inflammation

As with insulin resistance that is reduced when we eliminate damaging blood glucose levels, inflammation and the damage it causes is most effectively reduced when we stop introducing inflammatory substances into the body, either by changes in diet or environment.

You've just read extensively about omega-6, potent inflammatory agents, which have become the fatty acid cornerstone of the standard American diet (SAD). The single best way to reduce inflammation is to follow the advice on balancing omega-3 and omega-6 ratios, as described in *Optimizing Omega-3 and Omega-6 Intake* on page 151.

Some guidelines for anti-inflammatory eating:

- Avoid vegetable oils altogether. This includes corn oil, cottonseed oil, and soybean oil, which are some of the most common omega-6 laden oils in our diet today. Other culprits include safflower oil, sunflower oil, and generic "vegetable oil." It's pretty safe to assume that any commercially prepared salad dressing or mayonnaise is going to be loaded with some unfavorable combination of these. Even an "olive oil" mayo that I saw in the grocery store recently had more soybean oil than olive oil in it. And avoid margarine—it's one of the worst of all.

- Eliminate grains from your diet.

- Eat grass-fed beef, not grain-fed. In the same way that people who eat grains become unhealthy and inflamed, so do the cows that eat grains. Eating the meat from grain-fed cows only increases the omega-6 fatty acids in your body, thus increasing your inflammation.

- Eat poultry that is raised free range and allowed to eat their native diets.

- Eat eggs from free-roaming hens that are allowed to eat their natural diet, which includes grass, legumes, forbs,[1] seeds, and insects. Even if they're labeled "organic," I typically don't eat eggs labeled as coming from hens that eat a "100% natural vegetarian diet" because a vegetarian diet is not natural for a hen.
- Eat more fish, primarily the low mercury varieties. (Several online resources detail the mercury content of certain species of fish. For example, Skipjack tuna, also called "light" tuna, is typically low in mercury, presumably because the Skipjack is usually harvested before it has lived long enough to amass much mercury.)
- Eat plenty of (low-glycemic) organic green and yellow vegetables—they contain a host of anti-inflammatory compounds.
- Avoid processed foods whenever possible. Jack Challem, author of *The Inflammation Syndrome*, states it succinctly: "...Avoid any food that does not resemble what it looked like as it was growing or being raised."
- If you're effectively controlling your blood sugars, you're already avoiding the many forms of sugars and starches.
- If you can identify foods to which you are even slightly sensitive, eliminate them from your diet. Food sensitivities are extremely difficult to identify symptomatically because the onset of symptoms can be delayed by as much as thirty-six hours after exposure to the food. See Appendix K for information on a comprehensive food sensitivity panel that you can order.

By eliminating dietary causes of inflammation, you will probably eliminate the majority of the inflammatory factors in your life.

Reducing Environmental Causes of Inflammation

As discussed previously, many environmental agents can trigger inflammation and it's impossible to eliminate them all. We can, however, strive to minimize our exposure as much as possible. While relocating to a less polluted area may be impossible, equipping your home with an air cleaner may not be. If you walk, bike, or

1. Some examples of forbs are clover, sunflower, and milkweed.

jog in a smoggy urban area, perhaps you can wear a filter mask. It may seem silly at first but they're quite popular in Japan and increasingly so in the United States.

Replacing household cleaners that contain inflammatory chemicals with more natural (i.e., "green") products can substantially reduce inflammatory triggers. Even air fresheners are a source of inflammation for many people. It's better to attack an odor at the source than it is to constantly expose ourselves to the airborne chemicals in air fresheners.

When it's time to replace carpet, can you replace carpet with bamboo or wood flooring? Fewer airborne particles mean fewer triggers for asthma or other immune responses.

The books on inflammation listed in *Where to Learn More* contain additional suggestions for reducing exposure to environmental causes of inflammation.

Nutritional Supplements to Reduce Inflammation

The pitchfork-wielding, 3-inch lawyer on my shoulder wants me to remind you that any nutritional supplement has the potential to cause an unfavorable or harmful reaction. Do not modify your diet, take nutritional supplements, or begin an exercise routine without involving a qualified healthcare practitioner.

If your physician scoffs at the idea of nutritional supplements, perhaps it's time for a change. My physician has a list of every supplement I take and we review it at each visit. His biggest complaint is that I didn't start taking them 20 years ago.

If reducing environmental and dietary triggers are the first tier of a defense against inflammation, nutritional supplements are the second tier. Some other anti-inflammatory supplements that are worthy of your consideration include:

- Omega-3 fish oil (EPA, DHA)
- Niacin (primarily to reduce Lp-PLA2)
- Black cumin oil extract
- Kyolic® aged garlic extract
- 5-loxin
- Bosweilla
- Green tea extract
- Turmeric
- Milk thistle extract
- Bacopa extract
- Ashwagandha
- Zyflamend® [1]
- Protandim®
- Inflammasaver®

Vitamin D Levels

Vitamin D is crucial to optimal health. It is so important to so many systems in the body that I've devoted an entire section to vitamin D (which isn't actually a vitamin). See Appendix B for more information on vitamin D, including how to achieve optimum vitamin D levels.

---

1. Zyflamend®, Protandim®, and Inflammasaver® are commercially prepared combinations of other anti-inflammatory ingredients. You can, theoretically, duplicate the effect of these products by buying the ingredients separately, but these products are very convenient, backed by various amounts of clinical testing, and claim to contain optimized levels of their various ingredients.

Vitamin D Goal

Attribute	Goal	Notes
Vitamin D, 25-Hydroxy, blood level	50–80 ng/mL	Metabolism of vitamin D varies a great deal from person to person, making the question "how much vitamin D should I take?" far less meaningful than "what should the level of vitamin D in my blood be?"

EXERCISE

Few subjects spawn as many books as the subject of exercise (except maybe for diet and nutrition, that is) and I don't want this to turn into an exercise book. Like many other subjects, however, a number of misconceptions permeate advice on exercise, with many fitness trainers sharing the spotlight with dieticians in propagating backward and misguided information.

Why Exercise?

There are probably as many reasons to exercise as there are people exercising. For me, some of the most compelling reasons to exercise are

- Maintaining or increasing muscle mass (maintaining muscle mass is important as we age)
- Improving glucose metabolism (weight training to build muscle health is a great way to improve glucose metabolism and increase insulin sensitivity; be careful with weight training, however, as highly aggressive, stressful weight training can be an inflammatory process that becomes counter-productive to preventive health)
- Improving cardiovascular health
- Maintaining or increasing bone density
- Improving our general quality of life
- Just because it's enjoyable

You'll note that I didn't say that exercise was a compelling reason to lose weight. Read the works of Gary Taubes and you'll learn why exercising just to lose weight is a folly.

Consider Interval Training for Your Cardio

Cardio. Cardio. Cardio. One of the first things out of any health professional's mouth is that we need regular cardiovascular exercise to stay healthy and I certainly agree with that. The trouble with "cardio" exercise, however, is that many people do it wrong, according to Dr. Al Sears, author of *PACE: The 12-Minute Revolution*.

The exercise program that Dr. Sears advocates falls into the category of *interval training*, which is a type of exercise that mixes high-intensity exertion with low-intensity exertion. This is in contrast to traditional cardio where one traditionally warms up, exercises at a relatively constant and moderate level, and then cools down. According to Dr. Sears and other interval training advocates, traditional cardio causes the body to adapt to this moderate level of exertion by actually reducing maximum cardiovascular output.

Critics of traditional aerobic exercise argue that exercising the way most aerobics experts recommend actually retrains your heart to *reduce* its output so that it can operate more efficiently while performing traditional cardio (e.g., 60 to 70% of your heart's maximum age-adjusted rate), leaving no performance "headroom" to call upon if you need to exert yourself beyond what you normally do while working out.

Obviously, you need to consult your physician before starting or modifying any exercise routine, but if you're into cardio you owe it to yourself to do some research on the shortcomings of traditional cardio in favor of interval training. Many believe it's less pounding on the body, less time consuming, and far more effective at promoting cardiovascular health.[1]

---

1. When I ramped up my exercise routine, I first did traditional aerobic exercise. Then I switched to the P.A.C.E. interval training. The P.A.C.E. program produced much more dramatic results, lowering my resting heart rate far more effectively than traditional aerobic exercise did.

Additional Supplements to Consider

In addition to the anti-inflammatory supplements I talk about on page 157, there are many other nutritional supplements that have been shown to be beneficial. There are also many with claims that are not quite as substantiated. The best suggestion I can offer is do your homework. Don't add a supplement just because you read a headline or overheard someone advocating it in casual conversation. Treat adding a supplement with the same care and concern that you might take when adding a prescription medication. Ask yourself "what is this supposed to do?" and "what evidence is there that it's effective?" And know what side effects you need to watch for and what quantity is effective.

Also, when you decide to add a supplement to your diet, do so systematically (e.g., add supplements one at a time) so that you can carefully be on the lookout for any side effects.

Over-the-counter nutritional supplements have an exceptional safety record, but this doesn't mean you can afford to be careless.

That said, some of the many supplements that I've been compelled to investigate include:

- Cinnamon[1]
- CoQ10
- Vitamin C
- L-arginine
- N-acetyl cysteine
- Vitamin D (see Appendix B)
- Vitamin E (mixed tocopherols and tocotrienols)
- Vitamin K2

1. If you add cinnamon to your supplements, know that "Ceylon" cinnamon, also known as "true cinnamon" (from the botanical name *c. zeylanicum*) is reported to be the safest and most effective form of cinnamon, as opposed to cassia (*cinnamomum aromaticum*), which is also called "Saigon" or "Burmese" cinnamon.

Other Factors That Will Help

The biggest factor in achieving a healthier lifestyle is mindset. You must believe that the lifestyle choices that you make are the biggest influence in your overall health. We can't help our genetics but we can certainly control what we eat and do every day.

You also must be willing to challenge conventional wisdom. From "heart-healthy" vegetable oils (promoted, according to Dr. Mary Enig, as a direct result of their high profitability, not because of their healthful nature) to "healthy whole grains" (that are anything but healthy) to "just eat fewer calories and you'll lose weight," today's nutritional advice is fraught with misinformation, some of it well meaning and some motivated by pure profit. Add to this other outdated advice like the fact that merely monitoring our total cholesterol level (or even total LDL) is sufficient to define lipid health or that a simple stress test can tell you if you need to worry about cardiac plaque, and the guidance we're receiving grows even shakier.

Beyond achieving the proper mindset and addressing the factors I've already discussed, following are subjects worthy of your consideration as you and your doctor amplify your quest for improved health.

Thyroid Health

The thyroid and its role in overall health could fill an entire book. As hormonal creatures, our bodies are controlled by a dizzying array of hormones that influence nearly every single aspect of our metabolism.

From the perspective of cardiac health, the thyroid very significantly influences the types of lipid particles that the liver produces. Improper thyroid levels (typically low, or hypothyroid, levels) will cause the liver to produce unfavorable lipid particles (namely small LDL particles in great quantity and the harmful Lp(a) particle), thus dramatically increasing the formation of cardiac plaque. Unfortunately, many physicians (even many endocrinologists) diagnose thyroid insufficiency by focusing solely on the thyroid stimulating hormone level (TSH) while ignoring the levels of the thyroid hormones T3 and T4 (namely, free T3 and free T4).

TSH, you see, is the hormone that the body produces when it needs more hormones from the thyroid. If the body senses that the thyroid hormones are low, it produces TSH and the thyroid, in theory, produces more T4 in response. The T4 is converted through several means into the more usable T3 for use throughout the body. Most endocrinologists look solely at the TSH level and believe that if TSH is low, the body isn't calling for any thyroid hormones because the T3 and T4 levels are sufficient.

This completely ignores the dysfunctional body that is unable to produce TSH, despite an insufficiency in T3 or T4. Saying that because the TSH level is low, the thyroid hormones must be fine, is like saying that because a starving person has become too weak to beg for food, he must no longer be starving.

Rather than use the TSH as an *indicator* for the levels of the other thyroid hormones, it's a much better approach to measure and optimize the levels of the other thyroid hormones directly. In other words, if you want to know if T3 and T4 are too low, you don't ask TSH for its opinion, you measure T3 and T4 directly. It doesn't matter what TSH thinks; if T3 and T4 are low, they're low.

If this sounds confusing, don't worry. It's because it can be. The thyroid and its role in the body are amazingly complex subjects.

Studies have shown that most adults are suffering from low thyroid levels. The cause is not an established fact, but according to many experts, including Datis Kharrazian, the author of *Why Do I Still Have Thyroid Symptoms? When My Lab Tests Are Normal*, hypothyroidism is caused by an autoimmune attack on the thyroid. What causes autoimmune attacks in the body? If you read Chapter 4 on inflammation, you know that a variety of factors cause autoimmune responses in the body, most notably dietary factors like consuming omega-6 fatty acids and wheat.

One huge caution on optimizing thyroid hormones: I suggest you do so only with a physician who is skilled in *bioidentical* thyroid hormone optimization. *Bioidentical* means adjusting the body's hormone levels using the *exact same* compounds that the thyroid produces. This distinction is important because there are a variety of synthetic hormones out there, patented and promoted by the big pharmaceutical companies because naturally occurring substances (like human thyroid hormones) can't be patented. Not wanting to leave that potential profit on the table, the pharmaceutical companies patent synthetic hormones that behave differently in the body and then promote the drugs with multi-billions of dollars worth of marketing, aimed at convincing physicians that those synthetic hormones are as effective as the natural ones. I don't believe it and a great many physicians don't either. My advice is to avoid the synthetic hormones and work only with a physician who prescribes bioidentical hormones.

Hormone Balance

In addition to thyroid hormones, there are other hormones that may need to be optimized as we age. Here also I caution against synthetic hormone replacement, advising instead that you work with a physician who specializes in bioidentical hormone replacement.

What defines optimal levels of hormones is, of course, dependent upon gender and, to some extent, age. For men, the primary hormone is testosterone, with many over the age of 40 showing deficiencies in testosterone. For women, the primary hormone is estrogen, with deficiencies causing a variety of difficulties, including improper calcium metabolism leading to osteoporosis.[1]

Hormone replacement therapy is not without its detractors. Some will argue that it's harmful. Every such detractor I've seen, however, cites studies that use synthetic hormones, which is not the same thing as bioidentical hormone therapy.[2]

Remember, because pharmaceutical-influenced studies are typically a doctor's primary source of post-medical school continuing education, many doctors feel far more informed and comfortable prescribing synthetic hormones than naturally occurring, bioidentical ones.

Further clouding the issue of hormone replacement therapy, some studies supplement a single hormone (estrogen in women, for example) and when unfavorable outcomes are the result, argue

---

1. See Appendix U for more on osteoporosis.

2. In pointing out the absurdity of this comparison, many observe that introducing synthetic hormones that have never been part of the human body is *not* hormone replacement therapy—replacing lost hormones with the *same exact* hormone *is* hormone replacement therapy.

against hormone replacement. The flaw in this reasoning, however, is that all the hormones are connected. Supplementing one single hormone without optimizing the other hormones is just substituting one type of hormone imbalance with another. This isn't an indictment of hormone replacement therapy; it's an indictment of uneven hormone replacement therapy.

The message here is that bioidentical hormone replacement therapy is a highly effective tool for optimizing health and quality of life in individuals who are candidates for it. Unlike measuring our own lipids and changing diet to improve them, attempting to optimize our hormones without professional assistance is ill-advised. If you're interested in pursuing this, find an expert in bioidentical hormone replacement therapy and partner with him or her. Don't do it alone.

The good news is that more and more physicians are realizing the benefits of bioidentical hormone replacement therapy (BHRT). Searching online for *bioidentical hormone replacement* will likely yield practitioners in your area.

A positive side effect of finding a hormone replacement professional is that such a provider is also likely to support the other preventive health measures I advocate in this book.

Oral Health

Evidence has shown that harmful mouth bacteria can enter the bloodstream and bind with the plaque-forming agents, adding an additional bacterial component to the plaque. By limiting the bad bacteria in the mouth as much of the time as possible, we may be able to deter the bacterial component of plaque formation.

When we get our teeth cleaned, the bacteria are probably wiped out for the next 12 hours or so—once or twice a year. The rest of the year, the bacteria is being countered only by routine brushing and flossing, which is quite likely insufficient to touch every surface of the mouth and kill all of the bacteria.

While it's reasonable to believe that a traditional oral hygiene regimen is quite sufficient to keep the mouth and gums healthy, it's not likely to be effective at minimizing the constant trickle of mouth bacteria into the bloodstream that over time helps the coronary plaque flourish.

This subject is covered in great detail in Dr. Ellie Phillips' *Kiss Your Dentist Goodbye*, which, despite the title, is not actually a book about avoiding the dentist. It's a book that dispels some myths about oral hygiene and brings some very effective tools to bear in combating unfavorable bacteria that live in our mouths.

One thing I learned from Dr. Phillips' book is that the majority of sugarless gum is sweetened with sorbitol, a sweetener that's very cheap to make because it comes from corn. The problem with sorbitol is that in a significant number of people, harmful mouth bacteria can very quickly adapt to living off sorbitol, even more effectively than it does off table sugar, making sorbitol sweetened gum more harmful for many people's teeth than gum with sugar in it. The solution is to only chew gum sweetened with xylitol, which kills harmful mouth bacteria and to which the bacteria cannot adapt.

The Most Important Points from This Chapter

- Optimize your lipids, specifically your lipid subfractions.
- Control your blood glucose, specifically after eating.
- Watch your omega-3 and omega-6 intake by consuming adequate omega-3's and avoiding foods that are rich in inflammatory omega-6 fatty acids, one of the biggest sources being industrial oil products such as corn oil, soybean oil, grapeseed oil, safflower oil, and sesame oil.
- Don't speculate—use lipid subfraction analysis, glucose monitoring, and even postprandial triglyceride levels, if necessary, to monitor how your diet is affecting you.
- Reduce inflammation as much as possible by avoiding inflammatory triggers and adopting an anti-inflammatory lifestyle.
- Controlling glucose levels after meals is vital for everyone, not just diabetics, making an inexpensive glucose meter one of the most effective tools you can use in pursuit of optimum health.
- Exercise, done properly, brings many benefits.

One final note regarding goals: Don't worry if some of your goals are still vague at this point—the next chapter will address filling in any gaps you may have before you define a plan of action.

8

Plan of Action

There's a lot to preventive health. At times it seems as if I'm juggling a dozen plates just trying to address the many aspects I've discussed. Instead of letting myself be overwhelmed by it all, however, I find it helpful to view ill health as a set of interlocking cycles that feed upon one another. Viewing it in this way means the more of these cycles we can disrupt or reverse, the more we can potentially improve our health.

There's no single best way to go about this. Your plan of action will be influenced by many things, not the least of which is your personality. Are you the cautious type who will change one small thing at a time and carefully determine the effect of each change before progressing or will you fling open your kitchen window and hurl vegetable oil, flour, and wheat products into your yard, much to the dismay of your community association? Your personal comfort level and situation will guide you here. For example, it was easy for me to make radical changes overnight, eliminating vegetable oils and grains in one fell swoop, but even if you have decided to make radical changes, this decision may not set well with your family, who reach for their Whole Grain Cheerios, only to find that you've tossed them in the yard next to the bird bath.

Many people become excited about improving their health, only to be overwhelmed by it all and eventually give up. This is what gives rise to the adage "the perfect diet is one that you can live with." There's a great deal of wisdom in that adage. Yes, I know we're talking about more than a diet here, but you get the idea—it's important to be realistic about what you are truly willing to do.

On the other hand, don't sell yourself short and give up before you really give it a try. Radically improving your lifestyle may be difficult at first, but as soon as you experience positive changes (like more energy, better-fitting clothes, and dramatically improved checkups), you'll find that sticking with it is much easier than you thought at the beginning.

No matter your intent, trying to do all this overnight is probably an overly ambitious goal. It is, however, very possible to phase these changes into your life at a manageable rate, obtaining benefits along the way. I'm not saying it will be easy. To the contrary, it requires dedication and focus. It requires acknowledging that our bodies need to be cared for properly and that mainstream thinking is frequently not the answer. In fact, it's frequently a big part of the problem.

ADOPTING A PREVENTION MINDSET

One huge piece of advice I can offer is a change in perspective, switching from *fixing* or *improving* to *preventing*. As I talked about in the introductory chapters of this book, it's human nature to focus more on solving problems than on avoiding them altogether. In the context of preventive health, this is especially important because so many health products and foods are marketed to us as solutions to our problems that it's easy to forget all about preventing the problems in the first place.

While it's extremely useful to incorporate healing foods, spices, and lifestyle changes into our lives, it's typically just as useful (many times even *more* useful) to first eliminate the factors that are causing harm to begin with. For example,

- Omega-3 fatty acids are extremely beneficial; however, simply adding omega-3 to one's diet is far less beneficial if the person hasn't eliminated excessive sources of the damaging omega-6 fatty acids.
- Many foods and supplements have anti-inflammatory benefits, but taking them is far less effective without first eliminating the inflammation-causing substances from the diet and environment.

- Certain foods, spices, and medications will lower blood pressure, but don't forget to first ask "what's causing my blood pressure to rise in the first place?" and addressing those factors (and I can assure, it's very likely *not* excess salt in your diet[1]).

In other words, whenever you hear or read a news story or marketing piece that says "doing *x* will improve *y*," first ask yourself, "What's worsening *y* in the first place?" and take steps to correct that.

That said, let's talk now about implementing a plan of action.

Broadly Define Your Goals

After reading the preceding chapter, many of your goals may still be vague, especially if you haven't performed any baseline tests to fully assess your situation. For example, if you've never performed a lipid subfraction analysis, you may not know if your lipids are primarily small dense LDL particles or if you're producing the optimum number of larger, fluffy LDL particles.

On the other hand, you may already know from using your glucose meter that your postprandial glucose levels are reaching 180 mg/dL or even higher, compelling you to set a goal of reducing your postprandial glucose levels to 110 or 120 mg/dL.

You may know that you want as little coronary artery plaque as possible (who doesn't?) but you may not know if you're currently facing a calcium score of zero or one that's stratospherically high.

1. Moyer, MW. It's time to end the war on salt, *Scientific American*, July 8, 2011, p. 107.

An effective approach for finalizing the goals you set the previous chapter might be to review and categorize them into the following three groups:

1. List the goals that you can fully define at this point. For example:

   To minimize the progression of diabetes and the damage on my body, I want to reduce my postprandial glucose levels from their current 180+ mg/dL levels to no higher than 120 mg/dL.

   To reduce the damaging effects on my arteries of high blood pressure, I want to reduce my normal blood pressure of 140/100 or higher to be no higher than 120/80.

   To benefit the many structures in my body that depend on the proper fatty acids, I want to ensure that I consume no more than 3 grams of omega-6 fatty acids per day and that I consume at least 3 grams of omega-3 fatty acids each day.

   I'm convinced of the harmful effects of eating wheat—I would like to eliminate wheat from my diet altogether and to increase the amount of vegetables, nuts, and berries in my diet.

   To obtain all of the benefits that vitamin D brings, I would like to maintain vitamin D level of 50–80 ng/mL through diet, responsible sunlight exposure and, if necessary, supplementation.

2. List the goals that are less clear, perhaps because you know the goals but have no idea where you stand in relation to them, and define what you need to do to fill in the missing information. For example:

   I want my LDL particles to be the large, favorable kind and to have an optimal number of them but I first need a lipid subfraction analysis (e.g., a LipoScience NMR or Atherotech VAP) to know where I stand.

   I want to have zero coronary artery plaque but I need a coronary calcium scan to determine if I have any coronary plaque now.

   I want to minimize my levels of the harmful Lp(a) lipid particles but I don't know if I even have an Lp(a) problem. I need an Lp(a) blood test to know if I should worry about this heart disease-promoting lipid particle.

3. List the goals that are still very vague at this point, but that you don't want to forget about. For example:

   I know I need to exercise more, but I have no idea what kind is best for my needs or what my current condition would safely allow.

   I want to minimize inflammatory factors in my diet and in my environment, but without more fully assessing what I'm eating and what I'm exposed to I'm not sure what these things might be.

You'll note that I didn't suggest weight, body fat percentage, or waist size as a goal. These are symptoms, not problems. Instead of focusing on symptoms, address problems such as elevated glucose, insulin resistance, and unfavorable lipids and watch things improve. By all means, measure and be proud of what happens to your weight, body fat, and waist line, but don't make them your goal.

Now that you have a list of goals, ranging from very vague to fully detailed, what do you do? Simple. Get help to refine your goals.

Find a Partner

Everything is more fun with a friend, right? In this case, your friend should be your personal physician who shares your passion for preventive health and improving your lifestyle. I'm not talking about some crusty curmudgeon who is put off by all this newfangled thinking that's flying around the Internet and I'm certainly not talking about a fresh, newly minted physician whose head is ringing with the status quo attitude that permeates medical school today. Your partner should be a physician with a prevention-minded, whole-body approach who isn't afraid to challenge the status quo and who understands what Dr. Marcia Angell and Dr. John Ioannidis mean when they say that the overwhelming majority of what passes as research today is misguided and biased.

Unfortunately, there's no master list of physicians who "get it." Asking for recommendations from preventive health enthusiasts (there are plenty online) might be a place to start. I believe DOs (A DO is a doctor of osteopathic medicine) tend to take a more "whole body" approach than many MDs, but there are always exceptions. My personal physician, for example, is an MD who acts more like a DO. I've also found that calling a compounding pharmacy (a pharmacy that produces custom-made medications based upon physicians' orders) can often yield the names of open-minded physicians who are likely to be prevention-focused.[1]

When sitting down with your physician, you may want to

- Refine your goals and fill in the gaps, as described on page 172.
- Obtain the baseline tests necessary to assess your current situation (see *Establishing a Baseline* on page 130).
- Depending on your age and situation, you and your physician may want to pursue additional avenues, including:

  Testing thyroid and other hormone levels as a precursor to bioidentical hormone replacement therapy.

  Testing for food sensitivities (see Appendix K).

  Testing galectin-3 levels, a relative newcomer that is a by-product of macrophage production and appears to be a strong indicator for cardiac risk.

  Scanning for bone density, especially for females; the most commonly used test is dual-energy X-ray absorptiometry (DXA, also known as DEXA).

Join a Community

The support of a group of like-minded individuals can be a huge benefit when trying to make substantial lifestyle changes. Plus, as you start making changes for the better and begin seeing the many flaws in today's health advice, you'll likely want to spend time around people who "get it" and who won't look askance at you when you avoid wheat, say "no thanks" to corn, and turn positively

1. This is a subject for another venue, but countless blog posts by current medical students confirm that medical school instruction is still very centered on recognizing disease and choosing the best FDA-approved medication or procedure to address it. According to these students, discussion of optimal nutrition and disease *prevention* is scarce or absent altogether in today's medical school curriculum.

green when someone offers you something dripping in omega-6-laden vegetable oil.

For me, the single best community of cardiac-focused health enthusiasts is Dr. Davis's *Track Your Plaque* online community (www.trackyourplaque.com). This community is composed of some of the brightest and most determined people I've encountered. Presenting views from all walks of life, the Track Your Plaque members are unearthing new research and offering new insights every day, for the benefit of all members. Discussions range from sharing healthy recipes to delving into subtle biochemical mechanisms and everything in between.

Track Your Plaque also offers a set of tools for storing your test data and information about your diet, medications, and supplements, and if you wish, you can share this information (anonymously, under your user name, of course), to help members recognize patterns and trends that might be relevant to all. This is especially useful in looking for common factors in those members who show the most dramatic improvement in their test results.

If you have an interest in preventive health, especially cardiac health, I can't recommend the Track Your Plaque community strongly enough.

Establish a Baseline

Take a look at page 131 to see the list of baseline tests that I suggest you consider as a minimum. Additional tests that you may want to consider include hormone testing and food sensitivity testing.

If there are still items in your list of baseline tests that you haven't performed yet and your physician is unable to help, you may want to consider taking care of them yourself. There are a variety of online and storefront testing labs where you can perform virtually any lab test at a reasonable price, as I cover in more detail in Appendix S.

FINALIZE YOUR GOALS

Now that you've met with your physician to further discuss your goals, it's time to finalize them. If the two of you have addressed everything, then you're good to go. If not, you can turn to other sources of information, many of which I list in "Where to Learn More." These references should fill in any gaps you have in determining what goals are best for you.

Once you have established your goals, I suggest you find some way to list them clearly, either on paper or on a computer, so that you have a place to record subsequent test data to measure your progress against the goal. The tools on the Track Your Plaque site are wonderful, but pen and paper will work just as well if that's what you're comfortable with.

START MAKING CHANGES

Reading books about a better lifestyle is easy. Talking about doing better is also easy. Actually making changes is difficult. It's tough to walk away from actions and foods that are a familiar part of our life, even if we're convinced they've been doing us harm. It's even more difficult if we're new at this and may not be fully convinced that these changes will bring about the benefits that we're hoping for. This is something that might require a leap of faith: start living a better lifestyle and have faith that you'll see benefits. The changes may be slower in coming than you want or they may be different from what you expect, but they'll come. We really are what we eat.

As you start changing your diet, seriously consider keeping a food log to track everything you eat. It may seem like a pain but it can be very useful if you need to modify your diet in response to future lab tests. For example, if you find that your lipid subfraction suddenly takes a turn for the worse, showing dramatically less favorable particle counts or size, then you can take a look at your food logs to see if changes in your diet might be responsible. See Appendix L for information on some tools that could be useful. As you zero in on what's most favorable for you to eat, you can probably stop logging every little thing you eat and just continue eating the way that's working for you, but at the beginning, having the data at hand can be very useful.

At first, this strange new way of eating without grains and sugars can seem daunting, but a variety of wonderful cookbooks are out there. Take a look at Appendix R for additional information on some great sources of advice for keeping your healthy eating interesting.

Stop the Unfavorable

As I've mentioned before, often the easiest change one can make is to simply stop doing the things that are harmful—there's typically no preparation or elaborate investment involved. For example,

- Eliminate those foods that you should no longer consume, including all grains, especially wheat, corn, starchy vegetables, potatoes, refined sugar, and fructose, except in very small quantities in the occasional fruit (no fruit juice; it's the worst). Avoid all foods that your glucose meter shows to unfavorably elevate your blood glucose. Eliminate any omega-6 laden oils, including soybean oil, safflower oil, margarine, and cottonseed oil, by using references such as *The Ultimate Omega-3 Diet* and *Know Your Fats* to determine which oils are laden with inflammatory omega-6. Avoid as many processed foods as possible.

  This was the first step for me. Once I made up my mind to eliminate these things from my diet, it was a simple matter to replace those processed, fake foods, with grass-fed beef, truly free-range poultry, pastured eggs, and produce from local sources.

- Stop harmful behaviors.

  It should go without saying that smoking pretty much ensures that whatever else you do to improve your health will be ineffective by comparison. If you are a smoker and care enough about your health to have read this far, you don't need me to tell you that you need to quit smoking. Right now.

As discussed elsewhere in this book, certain people will benefit from moderate alcohol consumption, with most studies focusing on a glass of red wine. Excessive alcohol consumption, however, is ill advised for a variety of reasons, not the least of which is the disruptive effect on your liver's ability to produce favorable lipid particles and the ability of your pancreas to maintain effective glucose control.

- Remove as many environmental inflammatory agents as possible.

Add the Favorable

Nature abhors a vacuum, as they say. For us this means that as you eliminate harmful foods, something better must take its place. You'll undoubtedly replace some carbohydrates with better carbohydrates (replacing grains with vegetables, nuts, and berries, for example) and replace proteins with better proteins (replacing nitrate-laden, overcooked, processed meats with grass-fed beef, fish that is low in mercury content, free-range poultry, and eggs).

If you're "eating to your glucose meter," you'll also probably reduce your overall intake of carbohydrates, as carbohydrates are the biggest culprits in elevating blood glucose. When reducing overall carbohydrate intake, that void will invariably be filled by increased fat or protein intake.

Previously discussed is fat intake, arguing strongly that healthy (e.g., non-oxidized, low omega-6, etc.) fats are beneficial. The same is true for protein. There seems to be a huge range of protein intake that's suitable for humans. Personally, I don't advocate "high protein" diets that obtain the bulk of their calories from protein. Instead, I ensure that I eat adequate protein[1] and don't really worry about it. Some days I eat eighty grams of protein and some days I eat more than double that. I really don't worry about how much protein I eat, as long as I eat enough.

- Begin adding healthier foods to your diet, including healthier sources of protein, like fish, grass-fed beef, poultry, and eggs

---

1. There seems to be no single answer for what the ideal amount of protein is. The "old" standard used to be one gram of protein per kilogram of body weight and that seems to have given way to one gram of protein per pound of body weight.

from free-range hens;[1] fresh vegetables, berries, nuts, healthy fats like butter, coconut oil, and those with favorable omega-3 and omega-6 levels.

- Introduce the supplements that you and your physician have agreed upon, possibly including niacin, omega-3 fish oil, vitamin D, and some of the previously discussed anti-inflammatory supplements.

  I take every supplement that I've mentioned, sometimes alternating those with similar roles. And, of course, I include my personal physician in process so that I can benefit from his wisdom, as well.

- Begin exercising, as recommended by your physician.
- Read avidly. Take a look at *Where to Learn More* on page 253 for a list of books and blogs that were inspirations to me, or to those I admire. Read those. Then read the references that *they* advocate. Never stop learning.

Monitor Your Progress

As you replace unfavorable foods with favorable ones and as your list of supplements grows, it's important to monitor your progress. Admittedly, it's a delicate balance. A person with infinite means could drive himself crazy testing too often. A person not diligent enough could test too infrequently, leading to suboptimal results. And, of course, your health situation will influence how closely you choose to monitor your progress. If you're 25 with no family history of heart disease and your lipid subfraction analysis is great, you will likely be compelled to retest far less often than if you're 50 with a strong family history of heart disease, horrible lipids, and a 99 percentile coronary calcium score. As a general rule, I tended to test more often when I was starting out, and now that things like my lipid subfraction and my other indicators have stabilized, I test less often.

1. Real "free-range" hens, not hens that are cooped up in a box and are allowed to be called "free range" merely because their pen has a hole cut in it that allow some lucky few to wander outside for moments at a time.

Glucose Monitoring — I advocate monitoring your glucose level very closely as you build a list of which foods are favorable to you and which are not. Once you have compiled such a list of "friendly" foods, you'll typically not need to test your glucose after eating unless you're eating something unfamiliar.[1] Periodically, you can recheck familiar items to ensure that nothing has changed. And, of course, monitoring your fasting glucose is always useful because trends in your fasting glucose can reveal whether your insulin resistance is improving or worsening.

Now that I've identified foods that are favorable to me, I check my morning fasting glucose on a regular basis and every month or two I buy a container of test strips and test my glucose one and two hours after each meal for a few days or a week, just to keep an eye on things. These periodic "snapshots" are useful in helping make sure that my diet is still favorable in gauging the improvement of my glucose metabolism.

Lipid Subfraction Analysis — After establishing a baseline, retest your lipid subfraction periodically, more often if it was unfavorable to begin with and less often if was favorable. Personally, I believe even the most unfavorable picture warrants retesting no sooner than eight weeks, perhaps even 90 days after making significant lifestyle changes.

When I first started this process and my path was unclear, I performed a LipoScience NMR every eight weeks. Now that I've identified optimal foods and supplements for me, I perform an NMR every three to six months.

Omega-3 Index — Including the Omega-3 Index analysis with the baseline tests is very useful for determining how things have improved six months or a year later. Providing that your diet maintains a healthy level of omega-3 and omega-6 fatty acids, I wouldn't expect this value to change significantly from then on. After the baseline and the follow-up test, I'd probably test my Omega-3 Index every two or three years, just out of curiosity.

---

1. I'm talking about those who are *not* insulin-dependent diabetics, of course. If you're insulin-dependent, you should monitor your glucose level as recommended by your prescribing physician. A great reference book for insulin-dependent diabetics is *Dr. Bernstein's Diabetes Solution*.

Coronary Calcium Scan — How often you choose to repeat your coronary calcium scan will likely depend on the specifics of your condition. Typically, annual scans are advocated for those who have a worrisome calcium score, whereas a person with a zero score may choose longer intervals.

Postprandial Triglyceride Monitoring — If you want to take it to the next level, you could buy a home lipid meter and see how specific meals (or carefully measured quantities of specific fats) elevate your postprandial triglycerides. If you read the chapter on fats, you may recall that a small percentage of people produce very unfavorable triglyceride levels when ingesting significant quantities of fats. This is likely due to a defect in the way that such people break ingested fats into healthy lipid particles, causing their systems to be overwhelmed by a large intake. Depending on your condition and the nature of your lipid subfraction analysis, this may be an important tool for you to optimize your diet. No matter what your fasting triglycerides are, if your postprandial triglycerides are insanely high, then you're doing yourself a disservice.[1]

Magnesium — As discussed in Appendix I, you may want to consider monitoring your RBC magnesium levels to ensure that your magnesium is optimized.

RBC magnesium levels change rather slowly. For this reason, I measure mine only a couple of times a year. I also supplement aggressively with magnesium to ensure that my RBC magnesium levels are optimal.

Other Testing — Other testing that you and your physician may want to check on a regular basis includes vitamin D (see Appendix B), ferritin levels (see Appendix N), and a Comprehensive Metabolic Profile that includes ALT/AST (liver function) and a variety of other metabolic indicators.

I checked my ferritin level initially and found it to be rather high. I donate blood every sixty days or so and am confident that this will keep my ferritin from becoming excessive again. I'll likely check

1. I found the CardioChek home meter and triglyceride test strips to be very useful for this. The section *Achieving Triglyceride Goals* on page 136 talks more about the usefulness of postprandial triglyceride testing and offers my thanks to Dr. Davis for his writings on the subject.

my ferritin level annually just to be sure. I check my vitamin D levels two times a year, with one of them being early fall to ensure that my levels are high enough during the flu season. I also ensure that I check ALT and AST liver enzymes two or three times per year.

A Typical Day

The preventive health lifestyle I've described here may seem like a significant disruption to our daily lives, but it's not as onerous as it may seem. When I first started out, I needed to set reminders in my phone so that I would remember to take certain supplements or do certain things at specific times. Now, it's all second nature to me and my typical day looks something like this:

- When I first awaken, I take specific supplements that are believed to be more effective on an empty stomach. These include amino acids (e.g., l-arginine, l-carnitine, l-citrulline), and vitamin K.
- Later, after I've finished getting ready in the morning, it's time for breakfast. A typical breakfast might include free range, pastured eggs gently fried in coconut oil,[1] vegetables, and perhaps some avocado. Unlike most people's breakfast these days, mine doesn't include any grains, starches, fruits, fruit juices, or processed food of any kind.
- After breakfast, I take supplements that work better when taken with food, including a B-50 (B vitamin mixture), cinnamon, CoQ10, omega-3 fish oil, garlic, magnesium, potassium, and some probiotics.
- A couple of hours later, I drink a glass of water mixed with cold-milled organic flax seed. I include flax seed in my diet for the micronutrients, fiber, and alpha-linoleic acid (ALA), a plant-based omega-3. Even though ALA is very poorly converted to the more usable EPA and DHA forms of omega-3, I

1. "Pastured" eggs are eggs that I buy directly from the farmer who raises them and that come from truly free-roaming hens who eat a natural diet, including grass, legumes, forbs, seeds, and insects.

still consume it for whatever undiscovered benefits it may offer.

- In the middle of the day, I take a break and exercise. I'm fortunate to have a gym nearby and I can squeeze in a one-hour workout without too much difficulty. I try to include interval training for my cardiovascular health and moderate weight training for maintaining muscle mass and improving glucose metabolism. I *should* exercise seven days a week, but like most people my aim is higher than my reach. I average five hours of structured exercise a week.
- Following the workout, lunch includes a protein source such as fish, poultry, beef, or cheese. In addition, I'll include vegetables, avocado, nuts, and possibly some blueberries or a few strawberries. These, too, are locally sourced directly from the producer, whenever possible. (I try to avoid nuts that have been roasted, preferring raw and organic.)
- Following lunch, I take additional supplements, many the same as those that followed breakfast. Some specific to midday include niacin and some fat-soluble supplements like vitamin D.
- In the early evening, after my stomach is empty from lunch, I take another batch of supplements, primarily amino acids.
- Dinner is typically a recipe from one of Dana Carpender's low-carb cookbooks or from *Make It Paleo* by Bill Staley and Hayley Mason, followed by some after-dinner supplements, including more omega-3 fish oil and black cumin extract and other compounds featured in the book *Healing Spices* by Bharat B. Aggarwal, PhD, and Debora Yost.

While it's a bit more regimented than my previous lifestyle, eating and living the way I do now isn't really any harder. It's just a bit different. (Okay, it's more expensive, too, with the more wholesome foods and the supplements, but I believe that I'll pay myself back by avoiding expensive medical care as I age.)

Stay the Course, But Be Flexible

Give your body time to respond to these changes. There will be ups and downs. As Dr. Davis says in *Wheat Belly,* there will be real withdrawal symptoms when you give up wheat. Dr. Michael Eades has talked about the folly of "listening to your body" as you give up unfavorable carbohydrates, pointing out that just because your body cries out for something doesn't mean that it's making the right choice. It may take a few weeks before you have time to adjust to eliminating highly refined grains, processed sugar, and vegetable oils, and you will quite likely feel some withdrawal effects as you do so.

As things settle down, you'll almost certainly start noticing that things are better. You'll probably find that you no longer crave food every couple of hours and that skipping lunch is no big deal. Symptoms like acid reflux or other digestive problems may subside. If you have inflammatory or autoimmune conditions, you will likely see improvement from a dramatically improved diet. Soon the benefits of these changes will become apparent, and any inconvenience at making the changes will subside.

My suggestion that you be flexible is a reminder that there's no single solution for everyone. As you pay closer attention to your diet and begin watching your labs, you may need to adjust things. For example, if your HDL is too low, you may need to increase your fat intake. If your LDL particle count is too high, you may need to supplement with niacin. As time passes and your health changes, you may need to alter certain goals, strengthening them as your condition improves or relaxing them as your limitations require.

When you get to this level of attention and detail, you'll find that general advice about diet and nutrition can no longer do for you what your self-assessment can.

Prepare to Be an Outcast

I alluded to this at the beginning of this chapter, but if you really take to this newfound lifestyle of yours and start seeing dramatic benefits, it will alter the way you view the people and the world around you. You'll see ads for medications aimed at preventable conditions and wonder why the people of America don't do more to address *causes* instead of spending billions of dollars a year addressing *symptoms*.

You may find yourself biting your tongue every time you see a friend, colleague, or loved one wolf down a low-fat, grain-based meal, laden with vegetable oil, as they complain about having acid reflux or autoimmune disorders.

You may see friends and loved ones struggle with weight problems while they eat low-fat foods that constantly elevate their blood glucose level, ensuring that they live life as the "walking starving," trying unsuccessfully to lose weight.

Even your more health-conscious friends may not appreciate your one-upping them on matters of health and nutrition. Responding to their enthusiasm for fish oil with "yes, but do you track your daily intake of omega-3 and omega-6 fatty acids and have you ever checked your Omega-3 Index?" will make you sound like a know-it-all.

It's painful to realize that some people just don't want to hear that there's a better future available to them if they just abandon the current thinking on what's healthy and what's not. Many refuse to believe that they could ever get bad advice from a physician or from a "trusted" source like the USDA, the American Dietetic Association,[1] or the American Diabetes Association. In such cases, you may just need to silently watch them continue on their path.

"There's no free lunch," as the saying goes, and in this case it means that in addition to your improved health, the net result of all of this is that you may find yourself treading the very fine, and sometimes painful, line between helping people see the possibilities that an improved lifestyle will bring and making a pariah of yourself.

The Most Important Points from This Chapter

- Adopt a prevention mindset—first think about how to stop a problem at its source before you start treating symptoms.

1. The American Dietetic Association has recently changed its name to Academy of Nutrition and Dietetics.

- Establish a baseline so that you can measure progress in a real, objective way.
- Use the goals chapter, additional resources, and your physician to clearly define goals specific to you.
- Don't get tunnel vision on doing helpful things and forget to eliminate harmful things.
- Give your body time to adjust to the changes of an improved lifestyle.
- Monitor your progress regularly and make careful course corrections, always giving your body time to respond.
- Be prepared to see the world in a different light as your health improves and you see your friends and family struggle with preventable diseases.

Appendixes

APPENDIX A

CURRENT THEORIES OF CHOLESTEROL HEALTH

The current theories of cholesterol health are vital to understanding why there's so much misinformation out there because much of what we're told is good for us or bad for us is based upon these current theories, flawed that they are. To help weed through the dizzying array of advice out there, learn these two theories, including what's right about them and what's wrong. You'll be much more informed than if you just relied on sound bites or generalizations.

Here we go...

The story of today's cholesterol/heart disease model has a fascinating and frustrating history. Started by scientists in the 1950s who had discovered only part of the picture and fueled by politicians who wanted to take action designed to impress the voters (action based upon unproven research), today's theories on the cause of heart disease are fraught with gaping holes in logic and proof. The picture is further complicated by decades of shallow coverage by medical reporters, who try to fit a complex subject into easily digestible sound bites. When you factor in the economic motives of food manufacturers and pharmaceutical companies, both of which have significantly more money and political clout than they had 50 or 60 years ago, the truth about diet and heart disease becomes even more muddled.

If you sort through all the opinions and theories in mainstream thinking today, those theories can be reduced into two:

- Eating cholesterol (and saturated fats in general) causes heart disease.
  This is typically called the *diet-health theory.*
- High cholesterol levels in the bloodstream cause heart disease.
  This is called the *lipid hypothesis.*

At first glance, it may sound like these two theories are saying the same thing, but they're not. The diet-health theory draws a direct connection between eating fats and getting heart disease. It doesn't talk about what's going on in the bloodstream; it just says if you eat lots of fat, you're more likely to get heart disease.

In contrast, the lipid hypothesis doesn't mention diet whatsoever and simply says if you have a high level of cholesterol in your bloodstream, you're more likely to develop heart disease.

These two theories encapsulate the advice that you're no doubt already familiar with: eating fat, especially saturated fat, and having high levels of cholesterol in your blood cause heart disease.

Unfortunately, these two theories suffer from serious flaws and while it's tempting to simply discard them as hogwash and declare them entirely useless, I believe it's more useful to recognize that there are kernels of truth within each. By identifying what's true and what's not true about each one, we can appropriately apply them to our preventive health pursuits.

Diet-Health Theory: Eating Fats Causes Heart Disease

This theory took hold on the basis of two major efforts: 1) feeding high levels of saturated fats to research animals and studying their coronary arteries, and 2) looking at statistical models to find a correlation between saturated fat intake among certain groups of human populations and their rates of heart disease.

While animal studies are frequently very useful in studying how a certain medication, food, or environmental factor affects the health of humans, they're limited by physiological differences between humans and the animals being studied. For example, in the most famous animal study showing saturated fats to be dangerous to humans, researchers fed rabbits diets consisting primarily of saturated fats and then detected early signs of atherosclerosis in the rabbits when they were dissected. The problem with this is that rabbits are herbivores. They don't ever eat meat. As many before me have questioned, how is force-feeding animal fat to an herbivore lacking any mechanism for effectively metabolizing animal fat going to provide any relevant information about how that same diet will affect an omnivorous human?

The other way that researchers attempt to substantiate the diet-health theory is by observational studies. Observational studies are those in which the diets of large populations are assessed (typically by questionnaire or government statistics) and are studied against the rates of heart disease for those populations. By showing a correlation between reported saturated fat intake and heart disease, supporters argue that the diet-health theory is valid.

As you might have imagined, a large number of population studies have been done to address the diet-health theory. The most famous researcher in the diet-health area is undoubtedly Ancel Keys, whom one could argue ignited the entire "fat is bad" movement that began in the 1950s.

Keys produced two famous studies on the diet-health theory, one in 1953 and one in 1973. Both claimed to show a strong correlation between saturated fat intake and the rates of heart disease, yet both had serious flaws.

Critics of Keys' 1953 study, dubbed "The Six Country Study," point out that:

- Deaths that were attributed to cardiac arrest may not have been accurate. According to a group of Swedish researchers, death certificates during that time period were frequently incorrect. As many as half of the deaths reported as myocardial infarction (heart attack) were actually caused by something else.[1]
- Keys estimated saturated fat intake using archival data from the Food and Agriculture Organization of the United Nations

1. Lundberg, CD, Voight GE. *Reliability of a Presumptive Diagnosis in Sudden Unexpected Death in Adults: The Case for the Autopsy* JAMA. 1979;242(21):2328-2330.

(FAO), which showed only the amount of saturated fats available for consumption within a country, not what was actually eaten. As one critic points out, the amount of saturated fat intake will vary widely *within* a country, based upon a variety of socioeconomic conditions.

- Keys did not include data from all of the countries that he examined, only those that fit his diet-health theory. He had data on 22 countries, but he chose only the six that fit his theory, excluding the data from the other 16 countries. *Plotting the data from all 22 countries showed no correlation between dietary fat intake and death rates from heart disease.*[1]

Unfortunately, the second Keys study, published in 1972 and dubbed "The Seven Countries Study," fares no better. Critics of this study point out a number of serious flaws, including the fact that Keys had data for more than the seven countries that he included in his study—once again he excluded the countries that did not fit his predetermined conclusion that saturated fat intake caused heart disease.

The worth of Keys' studies is likely represented by the comments of statistician Russell H. Smith regarding the Seven Countries Study.

> The dietary assessment methodology was highly inconsistent across cohorts and thoroughly suspect. In addition, careful examination of the death rates and associations between diet and death rates reveal a massive set of inconsistencies and contradictions.
>
> It is almost inconceivable that the Seven Countries study was performed with such scientific abandon. It is also dumbfounding how the NHLBI/AHA alliance ignored such sloppiness in their many "rave reviews" of the study.

1. Yerushalmey J, Hilleboe HE. Fat in the diet and mortality from heart disease: A methodological note. *The New York State Journal of Medicine* 1957;57:2343-2354.

> In summary, the diet-CHD [coronary heart disease] relationship reported for the Seven Countries study cannot be taken seriously by the objective and critical scientist.[1]

Studies Contradicting the Diet-Health Theory

Not surprising are the countless studies that contradict the diet-health theory. Unfortunately, we don't typically hear about them in mainstream publications because the diet-health theory is still so firmly entrenched. A few of the studies are:

- A 1967 study in *British Heart Journal* examined more than a million employees of the India railway system and found that the group of employees consuming more than 16 times the fat (mostly saturated fat) had six times *fewer* heart attack deaths.[2]
- Two 2008 studies showed that the amount of saturated fat reaching the bloodstream is not a function of dietary saturated fat but is instead the product of dietary carbohydrates.[3]
- A study released in 2009 by the World Health Organization, historically one of the most staunch supporters of the diet-health theory, makes a dramatic shift from previous statements, saying "...the available evidence from cohort and randomized controlled trials is unsatisfactory and unreliable to make judgements about and substantiate the effects of dietary fat on the risks of developing CHD."[4]
- A 2010 *Journal of Clinical Nutrition* meta-analysis (i.e., a study that encompasses a large group of other analyses) showed that

---

1. Smith R, Pinckney ER. *Diet, blood cholesterol and coronary heart disease: A critical review of the literature.* Sherman Oaks, CA: Vector Enterprises, 1991. California.

2. Malotra, SL. Epidemiology of ischaemic heart disease in India with special reference to causation. *British Heart Journal* 1967:29:895-905.

3. Volek, JS, et al. Dietary carbohydrate restriction induces a unique metabolic state positively affecting atherogenic dyslipidemia, fatty acid partitioning, and metabolic syndrome. *Progress in Lipid Research* 2008; 47:307-318.

   Forsythe, CE, et al. Comparison of low fat and low carbohydrate diets on circulating fatty acid composition and markers of inflammation. *Lipids* 2008;43:65-77.

4. Burlingham, B, et al. Fats and Fatty Acids in Human Nutrition: Introduction. *Annals of Nutrition and Metabolism* 2009:55:1-308.

there is no substantial evidence that dietary saturated fat is associated with an increased risk of heart disease.[1]

The Lipid Hypothesis: High Blood Cholesterol Causes Heart Disease

The second of the two prevailing theories on cholesterol, the lipid hypothesis, doesn't attempt to address the source of cholesterol; it simply says that high levels of cholesterol (now revised to say high levels of LDL cholesterol) cause heart disease. As with the diet-health theory, the lipid hypothesis suffers from some serious flaws; however, the lipid hypothesis seems to be pointed more in the correct direction than the diet-health theory.

The Birth of the Lipid Hypothesis

There is a genetic abnormality that makes it far more difficult for cholesterol to enter a person's cells, thus causing the cholesterol to remain in the person's bloodstream, dramatically elevating blood cholesterol levels. This genetic abnormality, called *familial hypercholesterolemia*, affects about 1 in 500 people.[2]

When heart disease was far rarer than it is today, most young patients exhibiting heart disease were found to have familial hypercholesterolemia, along with the resultant elevated levels of cholesterol in their blood. This led researchers into believing that the elevated cholesterol levels were responsible for the early onset of heart disease.

Critics of this conclusion observe that there were just as many people with familial hyplercholesterolemia who were *not* suffering from heart disease. Healthy and without symptoms, these people had no reason to be noticed by cardiologists. Other critics note that prior to the middle of the twentieth century, there was no difference in cardiac mortality rates between those with familial hypercholesterolemia and those without. It wasn't until after the middle of the twentieth century that differences appeared, indicat-

---

1. Siri-Tarino, PW, et al. Saturated fat, carbohydrate, and cardiovascular disease. *American Journal of Clinical Nutrition* 2010;91:502-509.

2. Genetics Home Reference, a service of the US National Library of Medicine, part of the National Institutes of Health, an agency of the Department of Health and Human Services. http://ghr.nlm.nih.gov/

ing other factors (perhaps the modern diet of refined grains and vegetable oils?) are responsible.

Nonetheless, this perceived phenomenon gave birth to the lipid hypothesis that high levels of cholesterol cause heart disease. Other researchers quickly turned their attention to cholesterol in an attempt to substantiate this theory.

The trouble is, study after study showed no correlation between cholesterol levels in the blood and coronary artery disease. Studies that researchers believed would support the lipid hypothesis turned out to conflict with it. Consider these few studies from among many:

- An analysis of nearly 137,000 patients admitted to emergency rooms for coronary artery disease revealed that almost half of the patients hospitalized with CAD had admission LDL levels less than 100 mg/dL,[1] and 17.6% of the patients had LDL levels less than 70 mg/dL. According to the researchers, "a substantial proportion of patients presented with their first or recurrent CHD events well within the current guideline-recommended targets for LDL."[2] Amazingly, seeing that half the patients admitted for coronary artery disease have normal or below normal LDL levels didn't make the researchers think that they needed to reevaluate their theory. Their conclusion? They advised lowering the recommended cholesterol levels even more.
- More than 80,000 women from six different countries were studied for several years and found that there was no difference in cholesterol levels between those who had heart disease and those who did not.[3]

---

1. LDL-C levels below 100 mg/dL are considered optimal by virtually all mainstream health experts.

2. Sachdeva, A, et al. Lipid levels in patients hospitalized with coronary artery disease: An analysis of 136,905 hospitalizations in Get With The Guidelines; *American Heart Journal.* 2009 Jan; 157(1):111–117.

3. Jacobs, D, et al. Report of the Conference on Low Blood Cholesterol: Mortality Associations. *Circulation.* 1992;86:1046–1060.

- A study of elderly people from New York showed that those with *low* cholesterol, not high, had an increased risk of cardiac risk.[1]

Drug Companies: Championing the Lipid Hypothesis

Despite the glaring flaws in the theory, it didn't take long for the drug companies to realize that there was gold to be found in the lipid hypothesis. The trouble is, they first had to do what population studies thus far had failed to do: show that increased cholesterol levels caused heart disease.

Because observational studies had failed to show a correlation between cholesterol levels and heart disease, it became obvious that drug companies would have to prove this theory by using *cholesterol-lowering* medications to lower people's cholesterol levels and then show that those who had their cholesterol lowered were at a lesser risk for heart disease. If the drug companies could succeed in lowering cholesterol with drugs and then show a reduced rate of heart disease, they would reap a considerable profit in the form of medications designed to lower cholesterol.

The early studies with the first cholesterol-lowering drugs (fibrates) weren't very successful. In fact, many of them showed that the drugs actually increased the rates of heart attack and death. For this reason, drug companies quickly abandoned fibrates in favor of statins, which promised to be more effective.

Unfortunately, the statin trials didn't produce the stellar results that the drug companies had hoped for.

One of the most famous statin trials, the WOSCOPS (West of Scotland Coronary Prevention Study) trial, studied prevastatin's effectiveness on 6,000 middle-aged men. Five years on the medication showed that 1.6% of the non-treated (control) participants died of heart attacks during the study while 1.2% of the participants taking prevastain died of a heart attack during the same period.[2]

---

1. Krumholz, HM, et al. Lack of Association Between Cholesterol and Coronary Heart Disease Mortality and Morbidity and All-Cause Mortality in Persons Older Than 70 Years. *JAMA* 1994;272:1335–1340.

2. Shepherd, J, et al. Prevention of Coronary Heart Disease with Prevastain in Men with Hypercholesterolemia. *New England Journal of Medicine* 1995:333:1301–1307.

Put another way, if 1,000 men (not women, because as you'll read later, there has never been a study showing that statins are effective at reducing overall mortality for women) took this medication for five years, four fewer of the 1,000 men would have died from a heart attack, while the other 996 men would face the side effects of a liver-altering statin for a total of nearly 5,000 man-years of exposure.

Though a failure by any reasonable measure, this statistically insignificant 0.4% difference was nonetheless enough for the drug companies to claim success, thanks to some creative mathematics. You and I might think that reducing the rate of heart attack death from 1.6% to 1.2% would be considered a reduction percentage of 0.4, but that's not the case when interpreted by a pharmaceutical company. You see, creating big expensive magazine ads and journal articles that proclaim a 0.4% reduction in heart attack risk wouldn't impress anyone, so they had to find a much prettier method of packaging these results. What did they do? Simple. When citing this study, the pharmaceutical company didn't report a 0.4% improvement, instead, they reported a 25% reduction in cardiac risk.

How did 0.4% become 25%, you ask?

Because they didn't calculate the *overall risk reduction* of 1.6% minus 1.2%, which would be 0.4%. Instead, they said that because 0.4% is one-forth of 1.6%, the reduction was 25%.

Stated another way, if a drug trial showed that a medication reduced the chances of getting a certain disease from two in a million (0.002%) to one in a million (0.001%), the drug companies would report that their medication reduced the rate of disease by 50% (0.001 divided by 0.002), not 0.0001% (0.0002% minus 0.0001%).

This calculation is called a *relative risk reduction* (as opposed to an *absolute* risk reduction) and the drug companies were betting that most people would just notice the 25% and not really pay attention to how it was derived.

And they were right. Ask almost anyone, even many physicians, about the reduction in heart attack risk shown by this study and they'll say that the statins reduced the risk of a heart attack death by 25%.

Think about relative versus absolute risk the next time you hear that something "decreases the chance of [insert scary-sounding disease here] by [some percentage]."

After all, if the risk of getting a disease is 1/80,000, do you really want to spend hundreds of dollars per month taking the latest medication, with all its inherent risks and side effects, to reduce your chance of the disease to 1/100,000? Probably not. But people are far more likely to buy the latest whiz-bang prescription medication if they're told that it reduces their chance of the scary disease by 25%.

Study after study shows similar results for statins: Trivial or non-existent reduction in heart attack risk, typically inflated by using relative risk reduction figures so that fractions of a percentage appear many times more significant. Many studies even show an *increase* in heart attack deaths from statin treatment, yet these are rarely publicized.[1]

And that's only part of the misrepresentation of statins.

A big misrepresentation about statins is that they benefit women, which the research simply does *not* show. As published in the *Journal of the American Medical Association*, for women without prior heart disease statins neither reduce the risk of heart disease nor of death. In women who already have heart disease, statins *do* reduce the risk of death from heart disease but they also *increase* the risk of death from other causes (like cancer and stroke), resulting in *no overall mortality reduction.*[2]

---

1. Downs, JR, et al. Primary prevention of acute coronary events With Lovastatin in men and women With average cholesterol Levels: Results of AFCAPS/TexCAPS. *JAMA* 1998;279:1615–1621.

2. Walsh J, Pignone N. Drug treatment of hyperlipidemia in women. *JAMA*. 2004;291(18):2243-2252.

The fact that statins have never been shown to reduce a woman's risk of death is even revealed in some of the drug company ads, disclosed in the microscopic fine print underneath the smiling woman who advises other women to take statins. Amazingly, physicians continue to prescribe statins for women, despite the increased risk of dementia[1] and cancer.[2]

---

1. King, DS, et al. Cognitive impairment associated with atorvastatin and simvastatin. *Pharmacotherapy* 2003;23:1663–1667.

   Orsi, A et al. Simvastatin-associated memory loss. *Pharmacotherapy*, 2001; 21:767–769.

   Silva, MA et al. Statin-related adverse events: A meta-analysis. *Clinical Therapeutics*, 2006;28:26-35.

   Wagstaff, LR, et al. Statin-associated memory loss: analysis of 60 case reports and review of the literature. *Pharmacotherapy*, 2003;23:871–880.

2. Newman B, Hulley B. Carcinogenicity of lipid-lowering drugs. *JAMA*. 1996;275(1):55–60.

   Sacks, FM, et al. The effect of pravastatin on coronary events after myocardial infarction in patients with average cholesterol levels. *New England Journal of Medicine*. 1996;335:1001–1009

   Shepherd, J, et al. Pravastatin in elderly individuals at risk of vascular disease (PROSPER): A randomised controlled trial. *Lancet*. 2002;360:1623-1630.

   Matsuzaki, M, et al. Large scale cohort study of the relationship between serum cholesterol concentration and coronary events with low-dose simvastatin therapy in Japanese patients with hypercholesterolemia: Primary Prevention Cohort Study of the Japan Lipid Intervention Trial (J-LIT). *Circulation Journal*. 2002;66:1087–1095.

Appendix B

Vitamin D: An Emerging Superstar

We all hate the flu season. The fear of fever, chills, body aches, and missed work or school is enough to compel millions of us to get a flu shot every year, producing a predicted $4 billion worldwide flu vaccine market by the year 2012.[1]

What if I told you that the "flu" season was nothing more than the "low vitamin D" season, brought on by the winter solstice?

Such is the focus of the paper by Dr. John Cannell titled "Epidemic Influence and Vitamin D" published in a 2006 edition of *Epidemiology and Infection.*

Vitamin D, you see, is produced by our skin when we are exposed to sunlight. Many call vitamin D "the sunshine vitamin."

1. Health Industry Distributors Association • 2007-2008 *Influenza Vaccine Production & Distribution Market Brief*

When speaking of the motivation behind this research, Dr. Cannell states:

> Then I thought of three mysteries that I first learned in medical school at the University of North Carolina: (1) although the influenza virus exists in the population year-round, influenza is a wintertime illness; (2) children with vitamin D-deficient rickets are much more likely to suffer from respiratory infections; (3) the elderly in most countries are much more likely to die in the winter than the summer (excess wintertime mortality), and most of that excess mortality, although listed as cardiac, is, in fact, due to influenza.[1]

His research into influenza and vitamin D provides extremely compelling evidence that the flu season is due to little more than the seasonal decline of vitamin D levels and that correcting vitamin D deficiencies would bring substantial benefits.

In his influenza paper, Dr. Cannell and colleagues propose that vitamin D explains a number of observations regarding the flu, including why more flu occurs in the months following the winter solstice, when vitamin D levels are at their lowest, and fewer cases of flu occur after the summer solstice, when vitamin D levels are at their highest. The study also proposes that vitamin D explains why in the tropics where sunshine is prevalent, influenza is more common during the rainy season, why there are fewer winter deaths among the elderly in countries with higher levels of vitamin D consumption, and why children who are exposed to sunlight are less likely to get colds than children exposed to less sunlight.

It's interesting to note that vitamin D is not really a vitamin. It's actually a "protohormone," which is a substance that's converted into a hormone. According to the Vitamin D Council, the product of vitamin D metabolism is a compound that unlocks over 2,700 binding sites on the human genome—binding sites near genes that are "involved in virtually every known major disease in

---

1. *Medical News Today,* September 15, 2006.

humans." It seems obvious to me why a vitamin D deficiency would have far-reaching implications in our health.

Dr. Cannell believes so strongly in the benefits of vitamin D that he formed the non-profit, education organization known as The Vitamin D Council. The Vitamin D Council cites many studies showing that an overwhelming majority of Americans are deficient in vitamin D and, more alarmingly, vitamin D is a critical factor in a very long list of functions in our body.

Conditions in which the Vitamin D Council asserts a role by vitamin D include:

- Cancer
- Cardiovascular disease
- Congenital and neonatal disorders
- Infections and autoimmunity
- Mental health and learning disorders
- Respiratory diseases
- Skin disorders
- Women's health

The best way to get vitamin D is through responsible exposure to sunshine. This is because our skin converts sunshine into vitamin D ("responsible exposure to sunshine" means avoiding sunburn). The beauty of obtaining vitamin D through sunlight exposure is that the skin will never produce more vitamin D than the body needs, thereby avoiding any concerns about excess vitamin D levels. Most people achieve health-promoting levels of vitamin D with just ten or twenty minutes of sunlight exposure per day.

Before you start fretting about sunlight exposure, you probably need to know that the subject of health risks from the sun is yet another case of the solution being the problem. The two types of ultraviolet radiation in sunlight that are absorbed by human skin are UVA and UVB. The UVB portion of the spectrum stimulates our skin to tan (or burn) and stimulates the production of vitamin D. UVA penetrates the skin more deeply and is potentially more damaging than UVB. Unfortunately, virtually all sunscreens block the vitamin D-promoting UVB and allow the more damaging UVA to pass. As we continue to avoid the sunlight and/or slather ourselves with damaging chemical sunscreens that block only the beneficial sunlight and allow the damaging sunlight through, we see rates of skin cancer increasing and vitamin D deficiencies become epidemic. Yet the traditional medical advice continues to be "avoid the sun."

If your lifestyle or skin type prevents responsible sunlight exposure, the next question is how much vitamin D should you take? That's not easy to answer. Due to the differences in how individuals metabolize vitamin D, supplementing with vitamin D can result in very different results for different people. This means that it's far less relevant to ask "how much vitamin D should I take" and far more relevant to ask "how much vitamin D should a blood test show?"

According to the Vitamin D Council, an optimum level of vitamin D in the bloodstream is 50 to 80 ng/mL.[1] Many people have levels far less than this, largely because they're overly fearful of sun exposure.

Testing one's serum vitamin D level is simple and cost-effective, available online for around $60. Make sure you check Vitamin D, 25-Hydroxy and not the less useful Vitamin D, 1,25 Dihydroxy. The levels of vitamin D in the body typically change rather slowly, making blood testing necessary only two or three times a year.

If you decide to supplement with vitamin D, many professionals recommends gel caps instead of tablet or pill form, as the gel caps are more efficiently absorbed. And be sure to take vitamin D3, not vitamin D2. Vitamin D2 is derived from plants and must be converted by the body into D3, which is a very inefficient process. If your doctor prescribes vitamin D for you, however, it may be vitamin D2 because D2 is what the pharmaceutical companies patented and received FDA approval for,[2] so this is what they

---

1. Don't confuse ng/mL with nmol/L. The former measurement is traditionally used in the United States whereas the latter is typically used in Europe. If you're researching vitamin D studies, make sure you don't get the two units confused.

2. Remember, naturally occurring substances from the body cannot be patented. Hence the pharmaceutical companies convincing your doctor that their high-profit vitamin D2, a form of vitamin D that your body has never produced, is what your doctor should prescribe instead of regular vitamin D3.

advertise to your physician. If this happened to me, I would instead take the much cheaper and more effective vitamin D3.

Appendix C

The Different Types of Diabetes

The biggest diabetes risk facing today's aging population is that of Type 2 diabetes, also known as *adult onset diabetes*. Accordingly, this book typically uses the term *diabetes* to mean Type 2 diabetes.

Type 1 — Type 1 diabetes means that a person's pancreas has completely lost the ability to produce insulin. Type 1 diabetes usually appears early in life, though it's increasingly appearing in adults (see Type 1.5). Type 1 diabetes appears to be an autoimmune attack against a the pancreas, though nobody knows exactly what causes it to occur.

Type 2 — Type 2 diabetes used to be called Adult Onset Diabetes because it was caused by progressive degradation of pancreatic function and increased insulin resistance until the body could no longer keep up with the demands for insulin, resulting in an inability to effectively metabolize glucose. It's no longer called Adult Onset Diabetes, however, because more and more youths are developing this form of diabetes, undoubtedly because of today's love affair with grains, vegetable oils, starches, and sugar.

Type 1.5 — The term Type 1.5 diabetes, is characterized by the same sort of autoimmune attack that one sees in Type 1 diabetes, with the difference being that Type 1.5 diabetes typically presents itself in adulthood and destroys pancreatic insulin production over a matter of months or a few years (insulin dependence typically occurs within six years of diagnosis). Insulin resistance is typically present in Type 1.5 diabetes but doesn't appear to be the primary cause (the autoimmune attack appears to be the primary cause). There are currently two types of Type 1.5 diabetes, LADA (Latent Autoimmune Diabetes) and MODY (Maturity Onset Diabetes of the Young). MODY has been linked to a specific genetic anomaly.

Because diabetes comes in a number of forms and because of the variability between individuals, it's important to remember that not everyone's diabetes will respond the same way to dietary modification. For example, a Type 2 diabetic who is in the early stages of the disease and who is not yet insulin-dependent may slow the progression of the disease considerably through carbohydrate restriction.

On the other hand, a Type 1 diabetic, whose body is not making any insulin at all, will not see the disease improve through dietary modification. What the Type 1 diabetic will gain through carbohydrate restriction, however, is better control of blood sugars and a much easier time managing injected insulin requirements. This refers to Dr. Richard Bernstein's term "the Law of Small Numbers," which states that if the diet causes only small changes in blood glucose levels, then only small amounts of insulin will be required to normalize the diet-induced glucose rise. The result of these small changes in blood glucose levels means that any inevitable imbalance between blood glucose level and injected insulin will be minimal and therefore much more easily corrected than if one were ingesting a huge amount of carbohydrates and then trying to compensate with a large injection of insulin.[1]

1. *Dr. Bernstein's Diabetes Solution* does a much better job of covering this. I recommend the book for anyone who wants to learn more about diabetes and its management.

Appendix D

How to Check Your Omega-3 Health

Consuming omega-3 and omega-6 fatty acids in the correct amount is vital to achieving your optimum health. If you're like me, though, you don't want to just trust that what you're doing is working—you want to verify it. You can accomplish this easily by having your Omega-3 Index tested by one of the many labs that does so. The Omega-3 Index is a numerical score based upon the percentage of the two primary omega-3 fatty acids, EPA and DHA, in your cells, and it is a powerful indicator of how well you have optimized your omega-3 and omega-6 intake. (Omega-6 intake is relevant to the Omega-3 Index because omega-6 fatty acids will displace omega-3 fatty acids if consumed to excess, thus lowering your Omega-3 Index.)

The testing company I used is LipidLab.com, operated by Dr. Doug Bibus. LipidLab.com seems to be a relatively young company but Dr. Bibus creates a very detailed and informative report, showing an amazing amount of information on the fatty acids contained in your body. The Track Your Plaque community also offers an Omega-3 Index test that appears to be comparable. Both tests involve placing a spot of blood on a test card and mailing it back to the laboratory for analysis.

APPENDIX E

WHAT A NUTRITION LABEL DOESN'T REVEAL

Food labels are a great thing. Without them we'd be completely in the dark about what we're eating. The trouble is, even with them we're still somewhat in the dark about what we're eating. This is due to very effective lobbying efforts by food manufacturers so that they can disguise as much as possible the harmful ingredients that might frighten away the more nutrition-savvy consumers.

You might think that labeling requirements are pretty simple: The label has to show what's in the product. In a sane world that would be true, but sadly, the FDA's labeling guidelines are not always about accuracy—they're frequently a compromise between science and lobbying. For example, there are times when 0.49 grams equals 0 grams and times when 10%, 20%, or even 100% can be shown as low as 0%.[1] As a consumer, it's quite difficult to keep it all straight.

1. http://www.fda.gov/Food/GuidanceComplianceRegulatoryInformation/GuidanceDocuments/FoodLabelingNutrition/FoodLabelingGuide/ucm064932.htm

Here are some things to keep in mind when looking at a food label:

0.49 grams equals 0 grams — Food labeling requirements allow manufacturers to round amounts that are less than 0.5 grams down to 0 grams. If, for example, a product contains 0.49 grams of sugar in a serving, the label can say "0 grams" of sugar per serving. This is especially interesting when we consider the next point, serving size.

Serving size sleight of hand — The manufacturer gets to define the serving size. This sounds like a harmless practice until one realizes that defining a smaller serving size is often used to hide the presence of ingredients that the manufacturer thinks that the consumer may want to avoid. Many consumers will overlook the fact that the package contains 2 servings (or 2.5 servings) and notice only that the product contains "0 grams" of whatever they're hoping to avoid. Here's an example of how this might work against someone who is trying to avoid harmful trans fats, for example in a packaged salad dressing:

- Even though the foil package is clearly designed to be torn open and the entire contents poured over a salad, the serving size has been adjusted so that one foil pouch of dressing is said to contain 2.5 servings.
- Even though one serving actually contains 0.49 grams of trans fats, the label reveals that one serving of salad dressing contains "0 grams" trans fat, due to labeling rules that allow the manufacturer to round 0.49 grams down to 0 grams or to avoid listing 0 grams and simply state "Not a significant source of trans fats."

  A quick bit of math reveals that the envelope that the consumer believes contains no trans fats actually contains more than a gram of trans fats (1.23 grams, actually). Nearly 1¼ grams of trans fats doesn't sound like a lot, but for the health-conscious person who is eating a variety of salads on a regular basis, it could easily add up to a few grams of trans fats every day.

  So how to avoid trans fats altogether? Look at the ingredients and avoid anything that contains typical trans fats culprits, like vegetable oil and soybean oil.

Sugar isn't sugar — This is a huge one. Only monosaccharides (e.g., glucose, fructose) and disaccharides (e.g., sucrose, maltose) are included in the FDA's definition of *sugar*. Polysaccharides (e.g., starch) are not included when manufacturers calculate the amount of sugar in a product. This, coupled with some serving size sleight of hand, allows manufacturers to include a fair amount of sugar in a food and still label it *sugar-free*. A starch-laden "sugar-free" food can easily contain a dangerously high amount of sugar. Remember, the true measure of a food's impact on your blood glucose is what your glucose meter tells you, not what the label tells you.

What's the best way to calculate the amount of sugar in a food? Equate *carbohydrates* with *sugar*. Simply look at the total for *carbohydrates* and subtract from that total anything that's listed as *fiber* or as *sugar alcohols*. The result is what you should consider sugar. For example, if a serving of food contains 10 grams of carbohydrates, 2 grams of fiber, and 3 grams of sugar alcohols, the net sugar (carbohydrate) in the serving is 10 grams minus 2 grams minus 3 grams, or 5 grams of sugar.

By the way, sugar alcohols are a relatively recent dietary component and can typically provide sweetness without causing an elevation in blood glucose. This is because they're metabolized later in the digestive process, in the intestines instead of in the stomach. Unfortunately, this causes many people to suffer from gas or diarrhea after eating sugar alcohols. Also, some small percentage of people *do* experience a rise in blood glucose from sugar alcohols, often many hours later, which can make it difficult associating the cause and effect. Nonetheless, sugar alcohols can be very useful when preparing foods that need some sweetness and you would like to avoid the sugar.

100% is really 0% — This isn't a misrepresentation as much as it's a common misunderstanding. The common food label includes a column labeled "Percent Daily Value" that reflects the percentage of a component (e.g., fat, trans fat, sugar, carbohydrates) in the product. For example, the Percent Daily Value column may show 0% carbohydrates, which many people interpret to mean that 0% of the stated serving size is made of carbohydrates. The real definition of this column, however, is the percentage of a given component *in the typical daily diet of 2,000 calories*. This is a very different thing, indeed, especially when anything less than 0.5% can be rounded down to 0%.

I'll illustrate with an example. The government-recommended intake of carbohydrates is 300 grams per day in a 2,000-calorie diet.[1] This means that a food having about 30 grams of sugar per 30-gram serving would show 10% carbohydrate in the Percent Daily Value column, even though 100% of the serving is sugar.

Even in the face of these uncertainties and misrepresentations on our nutrition labels, I find it most infuriating that labeling laws do not require the disclosure of genetically modified foods. This is not a question of whether or not genetically modified foods are harmful—it's a question of whether we, as consumers, have a fundamental right to know what's in the foods we are buying. Food manufacturers, and by their legislative inaction, the US Congress, are quite clearly telling the American consumer that they believe we have no such right.

1. What's another word for someone who adheres to the government's recommended intake of 300 grams or more of carbohydrates per day? "Diabetic." Don't believe me? Buy a glucose meter and see for yourself what your blood sugars are doing one and two hours after a meal that contains that many carbohydrates.

Appendix F

What Your Lab's "Normal" Range Really Means

Many people, physicians included, think that the Normal range for a test on a lab report reveals the *healthy* range for that test. This, unfortunately, is typically not true. To define Normal, most labs examine the data from all of its customers for a given age group and list the range where most of their test values fall.[1]

While this may seem a valid measurement of what's typical, it's not a valid measure of what's healthy. You see, there are many instances where the entire population is declining. Countless examples include magnesium levels (most people are deficient in magnesium, according to Dr. Michael Eades), fasting glucose (most people over 40 have fasting glucose levels that are too high), and hormones (a great many people over 40 suffer from suboptimal hormone levels). In such cases, all being Normal means is that you're just as unhealthy as everyone else your age. That's not very reassuring to me. I'd much rather aim for the optimal range—the range that brings the best health. In the case where most people have unhealthy values, however, what is healthy is frequently outside of the Normal range.

1. For you numbers people, what the lab typically does is define the Normal range as two standard deviations from the age-categorized mean. This means that approximately 95% of the people in a given age group fall within the Normal range.

Unfortunately, many physicians are concerned only with keeping their patients' lab values in the Normal range, not in the range that promotes ideal health. This is probably due to a number of factors, including teaching that defines Normal as *healthy*, insurance companies that refuse to cover tests and treatments for a patient who is Normal, and possibly a fear of litigation if something goes wrong when treating a patient whose labs were Normal to begin with.

How do you determine what's *healthy* versus what's Normal? Answering that question is the subtext of this entire book—helping you distinguish between what's really healthy and what is mistakenly believed to be healthy.

APPENDIX G

NIACIN: USEFUL BUT OFTEN MISUNDERSTOOD

The best thing we can do to optimize lipid health is to eliminate wheat, vegetable oils, and sugars (especially fructose) from the diet.

For those who think this step is insufficient, however, niacin can be a very helpful ally, as niacin (also known as *nicotinic acid*, or vitamin B3) can be very effective in lowering LDL particle count, increasing LDL particle size, and increasing HDL.

The biggest problem with niacin is that it typically causes a skin flush that freaks many people out. Some even mistake the skin flushing for a heart attack or allergic reaction and go to an emergency room in response.

The niacin flush, though annoying to some, is completely harmless.

Much misinformation about niacin results from early studies in which people took very slow-release niacin, effectively trickling niacin into their bloodstream all day. Niacin is metabolized by the liver and studies have shown that continuous exposure to niacin can elevate liver enzymes, a possible indication that the liver is being harmed in some way. Obviously, anything that elevates liver enzymes is a cause for concern. The reality, however, is that niacin is not intrinsically harmful. Rather, it's just that subjecting the liver to niacin for 10 or 15 hours a day, as these early studies did, is a bad idea. Unfortunately, many physicians saw these early studies, decided that niacin is too dangerous, and have closed the door on niacin's benefits.

Studies (and there have now been many) show that introducing niacin over a period of a few minutes (instant-release niacin) or even a couple of hours (slow-release niacin) poses no risk to the liver. The prescription form of niacin, called *Niaspan*, releases niacin gradually to reduce the niacin flush and through its FDA approval process was shown to be very safe and effective.

The over-the-counter equivalent to Niaspan, called *Slo-Niacin*, has also shown to be very safe and effective in numerous independent studies, which is not a surprise because it's essentially the same thing as Niaspan.

There are other forms that release niacin much more slowly than Niaspan or Slo-Niacin and they should be avoided, in my opinion, because they expose the liver to niacin for too long with each dose. Some "no-flush" forms of niacin are not nicotinic acid but are really *inositol hexaniacinate*. I think inositol hexaniacinate is a useless supplement and while it certainly produces no flush, it has none of the proven benefits that niacin does.

The US Recommended Daily Allowance of niacin is around 15 mg., which is way too low to show the lipid-improving effects that we're talking about here. Most people who begin supplementing with niacin do so starting at 250 or 500 mg. per day and increase from there if they need additional benefits. Of course, it's advisable to involve your physician in any changes in your supplements, diet, or exercise routine.

Some additional cautions I've seen regarding niacin include:

- If you are taking a statin, your physician may advise against taking niacin or at least may want you to ensure that the two are timed to minimize their interference with each other.
- Extremely high doses of niacin can cause blood glucose levels to increase slightly, though studies have shown that this effect is minimal and temporary and the glucose levels will drop again.[1]
- High doses of niacin can cause a benign increase in homocysteine levels.

---

1. Goldberg, RB, Jacobson, TA. Effects of niacin on glucose control in patients with dyslipidemia. *Mayo Clinic Proceedings*. April 2008;83(4):470–478.

APPENDIX H

MEASURING, NOT CALCULATING, LDL

When your doctor performs a standard cholesterol test and tells you your LDL value, it's not really a measurement of your LDL; it's an estimate. When routine testing of LDL, HDL, and triglycerides was first started, it was relatively easy to measure HDL and triglycerides but measuring LDL was a bit more difficult. To solve this problem, testing labs calculated LDL based upon a formula derived by Dr. Friedewald from the National Institutes of Health. This "Friedewald equation" calculates LDL using the formula:

LDL = Total cholesterol – HDL – (Triglycerides/5).

The problem with this formula is that it is very far from perfect and doesn't reflect the actual amount of LDL cholesterol present. The Friedewald estimate is even less accurate if HDL is low (a common occurrence in today's population) or if triglycerides are high (also common) or if triglycerides are significantly below 100.

In fact, it's been reported that depending on triglyceride values, a traditionally calculated LDL-C value can show anywhere from 16% to 61% error.[1] Think of that the next time you hear that someone was put on a statin because of elevated LDL or the next time your doctor tells you that your LDL is "a little high."

What's better than a Friedewald-approximated LDL-C? An LDL-P particle count for one thing. As discussed in *Particles, Not Cholesterol* on page 35, LDL particle count is by far the most relevant factor when discussing the amount of LDL in your body and the associated cardiac risk.

If you really want to know your true LDL-C value, pay $50 or so and have it directly measured, not estimated. The test is available from the various online testing companies and is called "Low-Density Lipoprotein Cholesterol (Direct)" or sometimes just "LDL Direct." It's interesting to note that a direct LDL measurement, because it doesn't calculate based upon triglyceride levels, is unaffected by what you have eaten recently.

---

1. McNamara, J, et al. Calculated values for low-density lipoprotein cholesterol in the assessment of lipid abnormalities and coronary disease risk. *Clinical Chemistry* 1990:36:36–42.

   Snidermana, AD, et al. Triglycerides and small dense LDL: The twin Achilles heels of the Friedewald formula. *Clinical Biochemistry* 2003:36: 499–504.

APPENDIX I

MAGNESIUM: MOST OF US ARE DEFICIENT IN THIS VITAL NUTRIENT

Magnesium is a critical element, involved in hundreds of critical biochemical processes in the human body.[1] A deficiency in magnesium, a condition common today, has been linked to some alarming maladies, including elevated blood pressure, arteriosclerosis, osteoporosis, and in some instances, sudden death.[2]

Widespread magnesium deficiency is undoubtedly caused by modern farming practices that involve large amounts of potassium and phosphorus, which reduce the amount of magnesium that growing plants absorb. In addition, most modern water supplies provide far less magnesium than well water from decades past. As discussed in the diabetes chapter, magnesium absorption is impeded by elevated insulin levels.

1. In fact, over 300 enzyme systems depend on magnesium.

2. Rude, RK. Magnesium deficiency: A cause of heterogenous disease in humans. *Journal of Bone and Mineral Research* 1998;13(4):749–758.

According to Dr. Michael Eades, nearly every doctor checks magnesium levels improperly. Most check serum magnesium, which is not an effective measure of how much magnesium is available for use in the body. The magnesium that matters most is the magnesium that has entered your red blood cells. The only way to determine this is to get an RBC Magnesium blood test, available online for about $45. According to my research, most magnesium proponents suggest that our magnesium level should be at the very top of LabCorp's reference range for age and gender.

Magnesium is tricky though, because it has a laxative effect (that's how milk of magnesia works: it's the magnesium). There are many forms of magnesium (e.g., magnesium oxide, magnesium glycinate, magnesium malate, magnesium citrate, and magnesium carbonate), and some people are able to tolerate one form or another with different success. If you and your physician decide that you should supplement with magnesium, it's probably best to start with a low level of a single form and increase the dosage slowly, watching for a laxative effect and monitoring your RBC magnesium level as you carefully control your intake.

Appendix J

Why Be Concerned about GBHs and GMOs?

You may have noticed on food packaging containers references to the contents being produced with "no GBHs or GMOs" and wonder what that means.

The piece below by Howard Vlieger of the non-profit *Farmer and Ranch Freedom Alliance* explains what GBHs and GMOs are and why so many scientists, farmers, and consumers are concerned about the hazards they pose—hazards not only to those who consume them but to humans, plants, and animals exposed by indirect means.

I became aware of the Farmer and Ranch Freedom Alliance when I started buying organic and naturally produced food products and learned of the pressures that are being applied to the small, independent farmers and ranchers at the hands of big agricultural entities like Monsanto and ConAgra Foods.

If you care about preserving your right to buy independently produced, organic and free range foods, I urge you to visit http://farmandranchfreedom.org/ to learn more.

Thank you to the Farmer and Ranch Freedom Alliance for their permission to reprint this piece in its entirety.

Glyphosate: What Is It?

by Howard Vlieger, *Farm and Ranch Freedom Alliance*

Glyphosate is the active chemical ingredient in Roundup herbicide and many other generic herbicides that are designed to kill all plants, except those genetically engineered to tolerate the chemical. Glyphosate-based herbicides (GBHs) are the most widely used herbicides in the world. According to the US Geological Service, there were 88,000 tons of glyphosate applied in the USA in 2007, which is the last year they recorded this data. GBHs are used to kill weeds in preparation for planting in no-till farming systems, as well as during the growing season for weed control in glyphosate-resistant crops. Glyphosate-resistant crops, often referred to as "Roundup Ready" crops, are genetically modified organism (GMO) crops. Because the crops are able to survive applications of glyphosate herbicide, the farmers planting these crops are enabled to spray glyphosate several times during the growing season. This vastly increases the amount of glyphosate used, increasing the environmental exposure and potential residues in the food supply.

How does glyphosate kill a plant?

Glyphosate chelates (immobilizes) many nutrients, including calcium, magnesium, manganese, zinc, iron, copper, nickel, cobalt, and boron, in the plant. This nutrient tie up occurs wherever glyphosate is present, whether in the plant, in the soil, in the grain, or in plant residue. "Chelate" is a Greek word meaning claw or to hold. This chelation establishes a very strong bond that inhibits the availability of these minerals. Glyphosate holds tight to these mineral compounds and does not release them until the chemical degrades.

In addition to the chelating effects of glyphosate, it is also a very strong biocide. Glyphosate kills beneficial soil organisms, including Pseudomonas, lAAs and IPPs. In addition to killing beneficial soil organisms, glyphosate promotes the growth of opportunistic fungi in the soil, such as Fusarium, Pythium, Phytophthora and others. The actual mode of action for glyphosate killing a plant is disease. Glyphostae prevents the natural growth hormones and enzymes from moving throughout the plant, and the plant therefore cannot grow and it cannot defend itself against disease. So when glyphosate is used repeatedly on fields year after year, the weeds build up their defense mechanisms against disease(s) and the development of "super weeds" is the result. As this takes place, the rate of glyphosate applied each year typical increases significantly.

Are there any known side effects from glyphosate?

Glyphosate is a known endocrine disrupter and has been scientifically proven to cause birth defects and infertility. Dr. Andreas Carrasco and a team of researchers in Argentina studied birth defects in frogs and chickens exposed to glyphosate. His study showed the same skeletal deformities in these animals as he was witnessing in the children that were born to the mothers who lived in an agricultural communities where large amounts of glyphosate were being aerially applied to glyphosate-resistant GMO soybeans.[1] A team led by Dr. Gilles Eric Seralini also documented significant damage from glyphosate to umbilical cord cells from human infants. Glyphosate residue kills both the sperm and the egg at a half part per million and caused endocrine disruption to the cells at 2/10 of a part per million.[2]

Is glyphosate contamination or drift an issue?

Glyphosate residue was detected by the US Geological Service in the air, rain, streams and rivers in the state of Mississippi in the 2010 and 2011 crop growing season and also in Iowa during the crop growing and spraying season in 2011.

How many people believe that glyphosate is a safe product to use?

Probably most people believe that it is safe. At many stores, you can buy ready-to-use formulations of glyphosate to spray weeds around the house, driveways, or even in your gardens. The warnings on the containers do not even mention any potential ill effects.

---

1. Paganeli, A, et al., Glyphosate-based herbicides produce teratogenic effects on vertebrates by impairing retinoic acid signaling. *Chemical Research in Toxicology* 2010;23:1586–1595.

2. Benachour, N, et al., Time- and dose-dependent effects of Roundup on human embryonic and placental cells. *Archives of Environmental Contamination and Toxicology Journal.* 2007;53:126–133.

What does it take for the glyphosate residue to break down?

There is no known soil organism or bacteria that has been identified to successfully degrade glyphosate. When glyphosate begins to degrade, the metabolite, Aminomethylphosphonicacid (AMPA), appears. AMPA is even more toxic than glyphosate.

Do you really want to have something like glyphosate around the house or on your farm?

APPENDIX K

FOOD SENSITIVITY TESTING

Inflammatory reactions can be delayed by as much as 36 hours after exposure to a trigger food. Meridian Valley Labs, located in Washington State, offers an assay panel that checks the blood for sensitivity to 190 or so different foods. Unlike the past where sensitivity testing involved a skin scratch test and watching for skin inflammation, the new assays are performed directly on a blood sample and are far more accurate.

If your doctor will order a comprehensive food sensitivity panel, great. That might be the ideal way to have the test. If, however, you do not have a physician who will order the test for you, this food sensitivity panel can be ordered without a physician's request (providing you don't live in any of the states that prohibit self-testing). As you'll see below, the slightly tricky part is getting your blood drawn.

After you contact Meridian Valley Labs (http://meridianvalley-lab.com), they send a blood draw kit directly to you. You can take it anywhere for the blood draw. The challenge is that Labcorp may or may not draw the blood for you without a note or prescription from your doctor.[1] If your local Labcorp won't draw the blood without a doctor's note, you may be able to get your doctor to request the blood draw (or your doctor's office may draw the blood for you).

After you have your blood drawn, send the specimen in the prepaid shipping container back to Meridian Valley Labs for analysis. They'll send a written report to you in a week or two.

When I ordered the test, the total price was $257, including shipping and handling for the kit, but if you change your mind and don't send the kit in and request a refund within 120 days, they refund 80% of $247 ($10 shipping, from the original price, is nonrefundable).

According to one physician I spoke with, many people are very surprised at the food sensitivities that they discover from this test and that people experience fantastic overall health benefits from eliminating or drastically reducing their exposure to these foods.

1. Some LabCorp locations will; some won't. It helps if you have a friendly rapport with your local LabCorp and go in at a time when they're not very busy.

APPENDIX L

KEEPING A FOOD LOG

My wife thinks I'm slightly crazy, but I keep a journal of everything I eat. Every day. If I need to, I can open my journal and tell you how many grams of carbohydrates, protein, saturated fat, monounsaturated fat, omega-3 fatty acid, or omega-6 fatty acid I had on August 17, 2010. Or September 4, 2010. Or January 9, 2011.

Yeah, it may be a bit much for most people, but I'm not just amassing data. I'm charting a course toward the optimal way for *me* to eat. Once I have that figured out, I'll likely be far less obsessive about tracking every speck of food that I eat.

I've found the following tools to be very useful:

Cron-o-meter — This free, open-source food tracking tool is cross-platform (Mac OS and Microsoft Windows) and contains the US Department of Agriculture food database with thousands of food items. You can choose which specific macronutrients you want to track and you can create custom food items or recipes. The program is a little quirky to use and has a couple of shortcomings, notably its lack of export capabilities and the fact that the USDA database includes fiber in the carbohydrate totals (most people discount fiber when counting carbohydrates), which can falsely skew the macronutrient totals towards higher than actual carbohydrate intake.

http://nutritiondata.self.com — The nutritional data from self.com is rather extensive. Just ignore their opinion about what's healthy. They still have their heads stuck in the "fat is bad" nonsense.

APPENDIX M

OMEGA-3 FISH OIL: PRESCRIPTION OR OTC?

The most obvious source of omega-3 fatty acids is diet. Foods rich in omega-3 fatty acids include certain fish and free-range animals. Many people choose to supplement their diets with omega-3 fatty acid supplements derived from fish oil. In fact, the benefits of supplementing with omega-3 are so pronounced that GlaxoSmithKline spent countless millions of dollars producing a prescription medicine that's nothing more than fish oil. The prescription, known as Lovaza, is FDA-approved and has been shown to lower triglycerides and improve overall lipid health.

Unfortunately, many physicians are conditioned to trust only FDA-approved medications and unilaterally dismiss any over-the-counter supplements. The more enlightened physicians, however, realize that most of the over-the-counter omega-3 fish oil products are equivalent to Lovaza and will instruct their patients to avoid the horribly overpriced Lovaza. One cardiologist in my area has racks of Sam's Club fish oil supplements in his office, which he sells at cost to his patients so that they can save the expense of buying Lovaza, which he states is no better but costs up to ten times more than Sam's Club fish oil.

The news media has published some stories recently about mercury and PCBs in fish oil. When it comes to PCBs, I think this is an alarmist reaction. According to consumerlab.com, an independent testing agency:

> Virtually all fish meat and fish oil supplement will contain some PCBs. The samples chosen were oils made primarily made from larger fish (including shark) and fish "liver," which tend to have higher amounts of contaminants. To put the findings in perspective, total daily PCBs reported was under 100 nanograms for most supplements and did not exceed 900 nanograms for any. The FDA permits an 8-ounce serving of fish to contain about 450,000 nanograms of total PCBs, 500 times more than in any of the products. The EPA, using a more conservative approach, estimates that the average adult can consume 1,400 nanograms of total PCBs per day without harmful effects.[1]

When it comes to mercury, I'm more compelled by studies showing mercury concerns not to be true, including one by Harvard researchers who affirmed that levels of mercury in the fish oils they tested were not an issue.[2]

---

1. www.consumerlab.com

2. Foran, SE, et al. Measurement of mercury levels in concentrated over-the-counter fish oil preparations: is fish oil healthier than fish? *Archives Pathology and Laboratory Medicine.* 2003;127(12):1603-1605.

APPENDIX N

WATCH YOUR FERRITIN LEVELS

Having the right amount of iron in the body is crucial. Too much or too little can cause problems. Most everyone is familiar enough with iron deficiency to know that low iron levels can cause symptoms of lethargy and malaise. What many do not realize, however, is that the symptoms of excess iron can very closely mimic the symptoms of iron deficiency, often causing patients, and physicians, to confuse one for the other. Compounding this confusion is that the levels of iron in the blood do not always reflect whether someone is iron-deficient. This confusion is the result of how iron is stored in the body, using honeycombed storage molecules known as *ferritin*.

You can think of ferritin molecules as iron bank accounts—as the needs of the body require, the body constantly moves iron from the bloodstream into and out of ferritin molecules, altering the blood iron level without needing to discard any iron from the body. (In fact, iron is not typically excreted from the body through any natural process, with the most common exception being menses.)

Why does the body move iron in and out of the bloodstream, hiding unneeded iron in ferritin molecules? According to Drs. Michael and Mary Eades, authors of *The Protein Power Lifeplan*, the most common reason the body intentionally lowers iron levels in the bloodstream is to fight infection. This is because invading bacteria cannot live without iron and they die quicker. As a result, a test for iron in the bloodstream during such an infection-fighting time would result in the appearance of an iron deficiency, when actually the body has intentionally pulled iron into the ferritin molecules in an effort to fight the infection. If a person fighting an infection begins taking more iron in an attempt to "correct" this mistaken iron deficiency, she defeats the body's iron-sequestering efforts and likely makes things worse.

According to the Drs. Eades, there have been cases of well-intentioned medical workers going to third-world countries and testing people's blood and finding them low in iron. The helpful doctors supplemented the villagers with iron and shortly after found a sharp rise in deaths from malaria or typhoid fever. This is because the villagers' bodies had sequestered the iron in their blood into ferritin honeycombs to help protect the people from infection and when their iron levels were increased by the physicians, the infections ran rampant, often causing death.

The net result of excess iron being mistaken for an iron deficiency is that iron excess is likely far more common than we think, especially because many physicians look only at iron levels in the bloodstream and don't check ferritin levels.

We accumulate excess iron from well-meaning but misguided iron supplementation, excessive red meat, or by ingesting wheat products, almost all of which are enriched with iron.

What does this concern with ferritin have to do with us and preventive health? Simple—if you or I were to have a cardiac event or a stroke where a clot formed, a certain portion of our body would be deprived of oxygen for some period of time. During this oxygen-deprivation period, the ferritin molecules will rupture, releasing a flood of iron. When the blockage is cleared and oxygen returns to the iron-laden environment, the rapid oxidation of the iron will act almost like a violent explosion, causing great damage. Some speculate that the damage caused by rapidly oxidizing iron actually causes more damage than the oxygen deprivation itself. (Damage that occurs when blood flow is restored is called "reperfusion injury.")

Some speculate that a person's ferritin levels are a significant factor in how much damage is caused by a stroke or a heart attack. For example, two people having strokes that appear to be the same severity may experience very different level of brain damage, depending on their respective ferritin levels. I don't know how much evidence there is to support this theory, but I have elected not to allow my ferritin levels to become excessive, just in case.

According to the sources I've seen, an ideal ferritin level is the lower 20% of the laboratory reference range for age and gender. For example, if your lab's result shows that the "normal" ferritin level for your age and gender is 20–250 ng/mL, then this criterion would define an optimal level as the lower 20% of this range, or 20–66 ng/mL.

If your ferritin level is too high, what do you do? Simple: donate blood. Depending on how high your ferritin level is, a few blood donations spaced 60 or so days apart (or whatever the donation period is for your local blood bank) should lower your levels to the optimal range. If you are disqualified from donating blood for some reason, you can probably find a phlebotomist who would be willing to draw a pint of blood and discard it a few times a year, providing you have no complications that would prevent this.

APPENDIX O

EBT VERSUS CT

Coronary calcium scans were originally performed using a superior technology called EBT (electron beam tomography), which provides a more accurate scan[1] with even less radiation. Unfortunately, CT scanners are replacing most EBT scanners today because of the CT scanner's greater versatility and lower cost. If you can find an EBT scan center in your area, that's ideal; however, a CT machine (providing it's at least a 64-slice CT scanner, preferably more) is still a superb tool for having a calcium scan, so don't let the unavailability of an EBT scanner dissuade you from having a calcium scan.

Because the difference in technology between EBT and CT can result in slightly different scan values for the same scan, I recommend that you consider sticking with one technology (and the same model of scanner if you're inclined to go that far for consistency) if you're going to be repeating scans from year to year.

1. Greuter, JW, et al. 64 slice MDCT generally underestimates coronary calcium scores as compared to EBT. *Medical Physics*, 2007:34;3510–3519.

APPENDIX P

PURCHASING DIABETES SUPPLIES

Glucose meters are cheap. This is because the real profit is in the glucose meter test strips, which can only be used once and then discarded. If you want to know what meter to buy, you can consult consumer testing sources to determine which are most accurate and/or economical, or you can call Dr. Richard Bernstein's Diabetes Center at 914-698-7525 between 9:30 am and 3:30 pm EST and ask what meter they're currently recommending. (You may recall that Dr. Bernstein is the engineer turned physician who is responsible for pioneering the portable glucose meter for personal use.) People who are diligent in measuring their blood glucose can easily consume ten or more strips in one day. Finding economical sources of diabetes test strips is therefore very desirable. Two of my favorite sources are

- AmericanDiabetesWholesale.com
- Amazon.com

I buy from a variety of Amazon sellers, depending on which is cheapest at the moment. If you do, be sure and check the Amazon listing details, as sellers will sometimes sell test strips very inexpensively because they are about to expire. This isn't a bad thing, providing you can use them in time.

While most brick and mortar stores will charge nearly $1.00 per test strip, I've been able to find test strips online for as little as $0.33 each.

APPENDIX Q

SOURCES OF SUPPLEMENTS

I buy a lot of supplements from a variety of suppliers. This is in no way an exhaustive list, nor can I guarantee that they're the best, but I have experience with the following companies and they may be a good place to start.

vitacost.com — They have great prices and a very user friendly website. When I log into my account I can see all my previous orders and can build lists of items that I frequently order, both of which make reordering very easy. I can also set up items to ship automatically on an interval that I choose.

purebulk.com — If you're someone who wants to buy the pure powdered form of supplements like vitamin C, beta carotene, or green tea extract, consider visiting purebulk.com.

bulkfoods.com — Do you like spices? How about powdered jalapenos? Geared more toward food items than supplements, bulkfoods.com is a great source for common ingredients and is much cheaper than grocery store prices.

pureformulas.com — Another great site for supplements.

myspicesage.com — A wonderful source for spices and herbs.

APPENDIX R

FINDING GREAT RECIPES

I couldn't have made this transition to a healthier lifestyle without a selection of great cookbooks that help keep healthy eating interesting for me. One of my favorite cookbook authors is Dana Carpender, who has published several low-carb cookbooks featuring recipes that boggle the taste buds. She also has a website (www.holdthetoast.com) that's quite informative and entertaining. Another wonderful cookbook is *Make it Paleo* by Bill Staley and Hayley Mason. This lavishly photographed cookbook will make you hungry just looking at it.

Many great websites are available, which focus on using healthy, natural foods in their recipes. The following are some I recommend:

- elanaspantry.com
- paleodietlifestyle.com
- everydaypaleo.com
- nourishingdays.com

Be careful when using cookbooks or recipe websites, however, as it's unlikely that any of them will precisely match the way you have decided you need to eat for optimum health. One may be nearly perfect but not share your desire to avoid wheat, for example. Others may say that they're "diabetic" cookbooks but feature recipes laden with flour, polysaccharides, fruit juices, and other unfavorable ingredients. Some gluten-free recipes include very high-glycemic substitutes for gluten, like tapioca starch, rice starch, and potato starch, which just replaces one unfavorable class of food with another. Other cookbooks may feature recipes that contain more omega-6 fatty acids than you're comfortable with.

Whatever the source, make sure that you study each recipe carefully and adjust it, as necessary, to match your specific dietary requirements.

Appendix S

Ordering Lab Tests Yourself

Most people do not know that residents of almost any state in the US can order laboratory tests online (or at a storefront, walk-in lab, like *Any Lab Test Now!*), without going through their physician. Exceptions to this appear to be New York, New Jersey, Massachusetts, Maryland, and Rhode Island, which require a physician's order.

All of the online companies I've used have sent me to LabCorp for the tests, just like your doctor probably does, and thanks to the online companies' volume purchasing, the price I pay for the test done at LabCorp is much less than LabCorp would charge me directly (and is frequently cheaper than my insurance company's negotiated rate).

The companies I've tried all follow the same basic procedure:

1. Log on to their confidential website and choose the test(s) that you want.

2. Pay for the tests online, using a credit card or PayPal. This is the total charge. There are no other fees from them or from LabCorp.

3. The site provides, either via direct download or emailed link, a requisition slip that you print and take to your nearest LabCorp at your convenience and have your blood drawn. Because the requisition slip says that you've already paid for the test, LabCorp doesn't charge you for your visit or even ask for insurance information (if they do, just remind them that it's prepaid).

A day or two later, you receive an emailed link for you to log into the test company's confidential website and download your LabCorp test results. Easy as pie!

The two companies I've used for self-directed medical testing are:

- PrivateMDLabs.com
- DirectLabs.com

Prices from these labs are somewhat comparable, but do comparison-shop for possible specials and combination offers, which might make one vendor more appealing and affordable than others.[1]

---

1. I've also ordered from INeedLabs.com but they appear to have been replaced by MDLabTests.com, whom I've not yet tried.

APPENDIX T

OMEGA-6 AND OMEGA-3: RATIOS VERSUS TOTAL AMOUNTS

Be very careful when talking about researching healthy foods and their omega-6 versus omega-3 content. Many publications talk about the *ratio* of the two fatty acids to each other and not the total amount. While I *am* concerned about my daily ratio (I try not to exceed a daily 2:1 omega-6 to omega-3 ratio), I do so within the context of the total amount.

For example, you wouldn't want to have a 1:1 ratio if you were eating 25 grams a day each of omega-3 and omega-6. This would be bad for two reasons.

- Consuming too much omega-3 has been shown to increase LDL particle count in some people, a clearly undesirable effect
- Omega-6 fatty acids are inflammatory, so even if the ratio is good, too much omega-6 is still bad.

This thinking applies equally well when analyzing individual foods, too. For example, if you look solely at the omega-6 to omega-3 ratio, coconut oil's ratio cannot be calculated because there's no omega-3 in it at all, meaning 100% of the omega fatty acid in coconut oil is from omega-6.

At first glance, this would seem to make coconut oil a very unfavorable oil, when in fact it's one of the best. That's because a tablespoon of coconut oil has less omega-6 in it than a single almond. This, and the very high content of beneficial lauric acid, makes coconut oil an extremely healthy oil to use. Just don't expect it to provide you with any of your omega-3.

An inverse example is walnut oil, which has an omega-6 to omega-3 ratio of 5:1, which doesn't seem too bad, considering some other popular oils have ratios that are nearly 1000:1. Looking closer, however, shows that a single tablespoon of walnut oil has almost *7 grams* of omega-6 in it, more omega-6 than a person should have in a single day.

The message here is this: pay attention to the total amount of omega-3 and omega-6 that you consume each day, not just to the ratios of the two in the foods you eat.

APPENDIX U

OSTEOPOROSIS: THE TREATMENT IS A PROBLEM

Imagine your swimming pool is leaking significant quantities of water. Nearly every day you notice that the water level keeps dropping. Eager to solve the problem, you call the pool repair company and ask them to come stop the water levels from continually dropping.

You return home from work that day to find a note from the repair company stating that they've taken care of the water leak for you. Going into your back yard you see five garden hoses draped into the pool and running full blast. Rather than patching your pool, the repair company has simply run hoses from every nearby faucet they could find, flooding your pool with a torrent of water to stay ahead of the leak.

Would you think the leaking problem had been solved? Not likely.

This is analogous, however, to constantly gobbling calcium to combat osteoporosis.

You see, in people with osteoporosis, the problem is very rarely a deficiency in calcium. The problem is typically that the calcium is going where it shouldn't. Instead of going into the bones, the calcium one is ingesting is going most everywhere else: into the kidneys, muscles, joints, and even into coronary arteries.[1]

Instead of solving the problem of calcium going where it shouldn't, we simply gobble up more calcium because the marketing sound bites and the product labels tell us that calcium is healthy.

The reason that calcium is playing hooky from your bones is very likely because of a combination of factors that include vitamin D, vitamin K, and hormone levels.

The solution to preventing or reversing osteoporosis is not simply gobbling more calcium. It's much better to properly control where your calcium ends up. One of the best ways to do so is by ensuring that you ingest sufficient vitamin K, either in diet or via supplements.

Vitamin K's principal role in the body is the regulation of transport of calcium into the bones. Insufficient vitamin K has been linked with osteoporosis and calcification of the heart valves and arteries. There are two primary forms of vitamin K, vitamin K1 and vitamin K2. K1 comes from plants and, while beneficial, is far less bioavailable than vitamin K2, which is abundant in meat, dairy, and eggs. The K2 type comes in two forms, MK-4 and MK-7, and both appear to be beneficial, even though they differ in how rapidly they are consumed by the body.

Research also indicates that vitamin K2 is also produced by healthy gut bacteria, providing even more evidence that gut health is vitally important to overall health.

In addition to vitamin K, vitamin D is vital to bone health, as described in Appendix B.

I've recently discovered a nutritionist who appears to have devoted her professional career to educating people about the root

1. M. J. Bolland, A. Grey, A. Avenell, G. D. Gamble, I. R. Reid. Calcium supplements with or without vitamin D and risk of cardiovascular events: reanalysis of the Women's Health Initiative limited access dataset and meta-analysis. *British Medical Journal*, 2011; 342 (apr19 1): d2040 DOI: 10.1136/bmj.d2040.

causes of osteoporosis and how to address the condition without ingesting harmful levels of calcium or taking dangerous prescription medications. From the introductory materials I've seen, the *Save Our Bones* program, by Vivian Goldschmidt, MA is a comprehensive program of diet, nutrition, and exercise that reflects the latest in scientific research on osteoporosis.

Check it out at http://saveourbones.com.

Where to Learn More

I wouldn't know much about preventive health if I hadn't become a student of some of today's leading thinkers, people for whom the truth is far more important than grant money, popularity, or mainstream endorsement. I encourage you to study as many of these sources as you can, and then continue on to find additional sources of insight and inspiration.

Publications

Healing Spices
Bharat B. Aggarwal, PhD and Debora Yost

The Truth About Drug Companies
Marcia Angell, MD

Atherotech VAP References
Atherotech

Berkeley HeartLab Clinical Reference Manual
Berkeley Heart Lab

Dr. Bernstein's Diabetes Solution: The Complete Guide to Achieving Normal Blood Sugars
Richard Bernstein, MD

Excitotoxins: The Taste that Kills
Russell L. Blaylock, MD

Clean and Green—The Complete Guide to Nontoxic and Environmentally Safe Housekeeping
Annie Berthold-Bond

Inflammation Syndrome
Jack Challem

Inflammation Nation
Floyd H. Chilton, PhD

The Cholesterol Delusion
Ernest N. Curtis, MD

Track Your Plaque
William Davis, MD

Wheat Belly
William Davis, MD

Protein Power Lifeplan
Michael R. Eades, MD and Mary Dan Eades, MD

Know Your Fats
Mary Enig, PhD

The Oiling of America
Mary Enig, PhD

Nutrition "In the face of contradictory evidence: Report of the Dietary Guidelines for Americans Committee"; Volume 26, Issue 10, Pages 915-924 (October 2010)
Adele H. Hite M.A.T., Richard David Feinman PhD, Gabriel E. Guzman PhD, Morton Satin M.Sc. d, Pamela A. Schoenfeld R.D., Richard J. Wood PhD

Why Do I Still Have Thyroid Symptoms? When My Lab Tests Are Normal: A Revolutionary Breakthrough In Understanding Hashimoto's Disease and Hypothyroidism
Datis Kharrazian

The Great Cholesterol Con
Malcolm Kendrick, MD

LipoScience NMR References
LipoScience

Inflammation Cure
William Joel Meggs, MD, PhD

The Art and Science of Low Carbohydrate Living: An Expert Guide to Making the Life-Saving Benefits of Carbohydrate Restriction Sustainable and Enjoyable
Stephen D. Phinney

Ignore the Awkward: How the Cholesterol Myths are Kept Alive
Uffe Ravnskov, MD, PhD

Blood Sugar 101: What They Don't Tell You About Diabetes
Jenny Ruhl

Good Calories/Bad Calories
Gary Taubes

Why We Get Fat: And What to Do About It
Gary Taubes

The Ultimate Omega-3 Diet
Evelyn Tribole

Websites

Track Your Plaque Blog
William Davis, MD
http://blog.trackyourplaque.com/

Track Your Plaque Community
William Davis, MD
www.trackyourplaque.com

Wheat Belly Blog
William Davis, MD
www.wheatbellyblog.com

The Blog of Richard Feinman, the Other
Richard Feinman, PhD
rdfeinman.wordpress.com/

The Healthy Skeptic
Chris Kresser L.Ac
www.thehealthyskeptic.com

The Blog of Denise Minger
Denise Minger
rawfoodsos.com

Fat Head, the Movie Blog
Tom Naughton
www.fathead-movie.com

Chapter Reference Guide

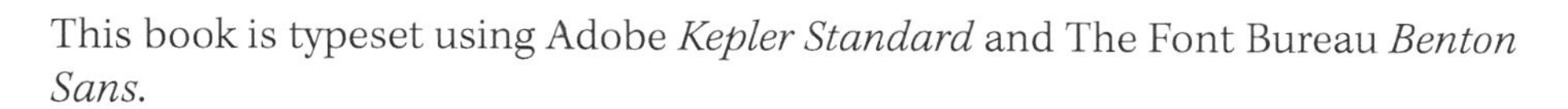

This book is typeset using Adobe *Kepler Standard* and The Font Bureau *Benton Sans.*

Named after the German Renaissance astronomer, *Kepler* was created by Adobe type designer Robert Slimbach, inspired by classic modern 18th century typefaces.

In 1903, Morris Fuller Benton designed News Gothic, a 20th century standard, which was redesigned in 1995 by Tobias Frere-Jones, based upon drawings in the Smithsonian. Cyrus Highsmith reviewed News Gothic, and in conjunction with the Font Bureau studio, expanded it into Benton Sans.

Made in the USA
Lexington, KY
13 September 2012